COUNTING

CARBOHYDRATES

CONTROL OF
PHASE II DIABETES

A PATIENTS POINT OF VIEW

By Winton N. Petersen

ISBN: 0-75961-669-8

This book is printed on acid free paper.

Address all inquiries to author, 6343 Safford Terrace,
North Port FL, 34287.

1stBooks – rev. 01/19/01

INDEX

PAGE

****

IMPORTANT NOTICE

Consult with your Doctor or Medical advisor before you make any change in your diet, exercise program, or medication.

This book outlines the action taken by one individual to control his Phase II Diabetes. It worked for him... It may not be for your condition.

Every case varies, and the knowledge of your particular condition is in the hands of your physican who has all information concerning your particular case.

****

Chapter 1

OVER 16 MILLION PERSONS IN THE UNITED STATES SUFFER FROM PHASE II DIABETES!!

I am one of those 16 million.

About two years ago, I weighed 176 pounds for my 5 ft 8 inch frame. My blood sugar count after fasting was more often around 180 to 210 than below that figure.

Today, I now weigh 151 pounds, my morning blood test is mostly in the 105 to 120 range, and I have reduced my 5 mg of glipizide tablets from 4 each day to 2 tablets per day.

NO, I DID NOT LOSE THIS WEIGHT AND BRING DOWN MY SUGAR COUNT BECAUSE I WENT ON A WEIGHT LOSS DIET. IT ALL HAPPENED WHEN I STARTED <u>COUNTING CARBOHYDRATES!</u>

WHAT ARE CARBOHYDRATES?

Most people are not aware of the fact that Carbohydrates that are not used immediately are stored by the body as fats!

From various sources I have obtained the following information concerning Carbohydrates:

Carbohydrates: Foods. These contain only carbon combined with hydrogen and oxygen such as sugars, starch, and cellulose. 98% of animal carbohydrates is digested. 96% of vegetable carbohydrates is digested.

Classification: Starches - Starch does not remain in the body as starch but is transformed or converted into sugar. They form fat in the body and produce heat and energy in the body.

Function: with the exception of cellulose, to provide energy and heat. **Excess is stored in the body as fat.** and a small amount as glycogen is stored in the liver for future use.

You will see from the above why such items as grains, potatoes, rice, Pasta, etc. (which are considered as good nourishment for those without diabetes,) care must be taken to take in only small servings for those with the ailment.

This book will show you how I did it and illustrate methods for you to easily follow the same program. I am addressing those of you that know that you are phase II diabetics and want to do the most for yourself in living with this ailment.

1

STRANGE AS IT MAY SEEM, WHILE IT IS A DIET THAT WOULD BE PRESCRIBED FOR A PHASE II DIABETIC, IT IS ALSO A HEALTHY DIET FOR ANYONE CONCERNED ABOUT A WEIGHT PROBLEM!!

Not all Phase II diabetics know that they have the disease! There are few physical signs that you have it until it has taken a toll on your body.

It can be easily detected with a blood test however. If there is anyone in your family that has had diabetes, (it is often hereditary), I advise you to have one performed as soon as possible.

Many organizations in your area perform this test free of charge so if you are reluctant to go to a doctor, check with your local newspapers for time and locations where these free tests are given. It only takes a pin prick and the results are known to you within a minute.

I am not about to attempt to override the advise of your doctor what will work for you. He is, of course, your first line of defense against this disease. However, he can only tell you what is best for you and prescribe the necessary medications to help fight your affliction.

It is up to you to adhere to his advise and to determine what works best for you in your dieting - exercise - and attitude. It worked for me, It could work for you!!

I was diagnosed with diabetes when I was 64. Since that time and until I reached my present age of 78, I have had to make adjustments in order to keep my condition under control.

Many times, it has not been successful, nor has it been pleasant, but all in all, I feel that now I have hit on a system that works for me, and allows me to perform all the things that I have been doing all my life. It does not interfere with my working a part time job, it does not stop me from traveling, climbing mountain trails, or playing with my grandchildren.

This book will not have a lot of information concerning the causes, or the effects of the ailment. Visit your local Library to locate any number of books covering the subject of diabetes. You are sure to find one that gives you the information you wish to receive.

Most illustrations here show the desired results of my own use of COUNTING CARBOHYDRATES, yet equally good results have been achieved by many of my friends and aquaintances who have asked me for copies of the book. Most are diabetics, but in some cases, they have used it to help maintain weight control.

The wife of one of my friends called me frantically one evening asking me to come over to take her husband's blood sugar count which had suddenly soared to over 220 pts.

He could not point to any particular reason for it, but he asked for a copy of my book to help him control the situation. With a sore on his foot that refused to heal he and his wife were very much concerned.

It also worked for him. He is back to work as a part time employee at a store, his blood count is down below 110, and his weight has gone from 210 pounds to 181.

Some of the credit must be given to his wife who watches his diet religiously...and in the process has also lost much weight while following the same food eating plan.

TAKE CONTROL! This is what you must do.

Don't expect your wife to prepare the meals and tell you what and when you should eat.

Don't alibi about not having time for exercise - that you are too old - that too many persons are preparing food you should not eat. The slogan, **"Just Say No"** used in fighting the use of Drugs pertains here as well.

And don't feel that just because you fall off the diet or cheat a little here and there that you have failed. We all do it, and with this ailment, it does not condemn you to a stay in the hospital or instant death. Actually, it is a matter of choices. No longer are you sentenced to a life time of denial of the food that you love. If you crave ice cream - you can have it. You want that piece of chocolate candy, go ahead and eat it, but somewhere, you are going to have to give up some other food loaded with Carbohydrates to allow you this luxury.

A class that I recently attended, the dietician gave this illustration: "You want a piece of cherry pie? OK, eat it, that is your mealtime allowance of Carbohydrates and you can't eat anything else with carbohydrates until your next meal."

CARBOHYDRATES!! Controlling my intake has worked well for me. Give it a try, and see if you can not obtain equally as great results as I have found.

Chapter 2

Why do some of us get diabetes and others don't?

Heredity is usually the big determining factor. My mother had it in her early 40's but as was the case in 1930 and 1940, it was never diagnosed. Treatment was not begun until she was in her late 50's, and by then the damage from excess blood sugar had been done.
She died when she was 63 yrs old following a stroke, partial blindness, and kidney failure.

My Dad faired slightly better when he developed phase II diabetes when he reached 62. Even at that point, he was required to take insulin, (the tablet treatment had not yet been developed at that date) but here again he found it difficult to adhere to the prescribed diet of that day.

His demise was when his foot became infected while cleaning up a sewer backup in the basement of his home. He had pared a corn too far leaving an open sore which later developed into gangrene. This required amputation above the knee.

Dispite this handicap he reached the age of 79 when he died of a heart attack.

With this background I should have been aware of the possibility of developing diabetes, yet it was not determined until I went to a VA clinic for stomach pains, was diagnosed with an ulcer, and at the end of the doctor visit he stated, "Oh, and by the way, you are diabetic."

Shocked? You bet. I think he could have said it a little more diplomatically, but it got me into action right away. I was told to see my own doctor to receive treatment.

I had recently retired as a letter carrier for the Postal Service, and I feel that the great amount of exercise required to deliver the mail held back the development of the disease until it showed up at the VA clinic.

The first visit to the family doctor, I received a 1500 calorie diet with all the exchanges, all the amounts of each item allowed, wt. limits etc. which made it almost impossible to follow.

I tried to follow them as closely as possible and for a time I was successful in holding down my blood sugar to a level that was an acceptable figure to my doctor. Testing was usually done once a month at a free Senior service location and approximately once every 3 months at my doctor's office.

Then my blood sugar began to climb. As it did, glipizide tablets were added to my intake. First 1 and 1/2 pills, then two, followed by three, and finally four. Again my count got up close to the 200 point mark when I decided I had to take my diet and exercise program more seriously.

I knew from my high school education that all Carbohydrates turn to sugar! So my logic said, why not count my carbohydrate intake, and forget about all the other factors on my 1500 calorie diet? I wasn't living up to it anyway because it was too confusing, so why not limit myself to approx. 50 grams of Carbohydrates per meal and see if it would bring down my sugar count?

I was now on a 1500 Calorie diet that allowed me 155 grams of Carbohydrates, so divided by 3 meals per day, I could consume 45 grams at each meal, and still have 20 grams for in-between snacks.

Soon after I attended classes concerning the control of diabetes and found out that the Medical Profession in 1994 had reached the same conclusion! They advocate the counting of Carbohydrates in foods - limited by the prescribed diet of your doctor - (1200 calorie, 1500 calorie, 1800 calorie etc.)

Unless you also have other limiting difficulties such as high cholesterol, high blood pressure, heart problems, etc. that require other dietary control, this makes living with this form of diet much easier.

The old method of food exchanges were not only confusing, but extremely time consuming to figure out!

I am sure that most of the other phase II diabetics reached the same conclusion and either took to "guessing" what to eat or abandoning the diet entirely.

Just as a diet does not work the same for all persons, perhaps your results may be different from mine, but it is worth a try. In most cases failure is due, not to the diet plan, but due to the failure of the individual to adhere to the limitations set forth in the diet.

Chapter 3

In order for you to keep a good record as to what you are eating and proper amounts, you should purchase a blood monitoring unit.

Since blood sugar levels change often during the day and night depending on the amount of carbohydrates or sugars entering the body, the only way you are going to know what is right for you as far as size of portions and what form of food you are eating is to take samples regularly.

I take a sample every morning shortly after rising from bed. This gives me an idea of what my average is and if I find that it changes to any great degree, I check to see what I had eaten the evening before that might have caused it to rise dramatically or even fall in some cases.

We are in the habit of eating out after dances on Friday nights, and sometimes the restaurant chosen does not have food available that are to the best interest of a diabetic.

This night Dunkin Donuts was the selected place so I said, what the heck, if I am going to cheat I might as well go whole hog. I chose an apple fritter...and not exactly a small one. The next morning's reading was 196, where my normal was usually below 120. Needless to say, a fritter will no longer be one of my choices as food. Without testing equipment, I would not know of this dramatic swing and most likely would go on choosing the wrong item.

Granted, the strips used for testing are expensive. (slightly under $1.00 each in most units), but with the help of medical insurance and now the recent approval of medicare coverage to pay for diabetic supplies, there is really no reason for not obtaining this necessary equipment.

Drugstores often have promotions of testing equipment in which huge discounts or rebates are given for the blood glucose monitoring systems.

All units do not use the same type of test strips, so purchase of their brand of strips is required for use in their testing equipment. This is where they make their money - hence the almost "Free" units.

Chapter 4

Determining amount of carbohydrates in foods

Over a period of time, I have collected the **Nutrition Facts** shown on all packaged food products presently being sold in stores. This is a Federal law that this be shown and is invaluable for one who must keep track of values of such items as:

Carbohydrates	**Fat content**
Sugar	**Cholesterol**
Sodium (Salt)	**Proteins**

WHEN CHECKING ON CARBOHYDRATE CONTENT, REMEMBER THAT THE TOTAL CARBOHYDRATE FIGURE INCLUDES THE SUGAR CONTENT. DO NOT ADD THE SUGAR GRAM FIGURE TO IT, AS IT IS ALREADY INCLUDED IN THE FIGURE.

An example of this is:
Reg. Vanilla Ice Cream contains 16 Grams of Total Carb.
The label will show 14 grams of sugar.
The 16 grams of Total Carb. INCLUDES those 14 grams.

While on the subject of Ice Cream, sure, I eat it. Portion size is 1/ 2 cup...but I do not measure this every time. I did it once and then estimate how much it is in a container. In most cases I possibly go over the portion size, but not excessively. As a guide, 2 level ice cream scoops is approx. 1/2 cup.

Don't be surprised when I tell you that I usually eat at least one such dish each day. In fact, I normally have some sort of dessert with each meal, other than ice cream it may be jello with cool whip and possibly a half of a banana in it - a dish of cook & serve chocolate sugar free pudding - or a couple of cookies.

Sure, I add in the number of grams of Carb. in the serving as part of my meal, and what I eat is determined by the total Carb. in the meal I have just eaten. If my meal is close to the 50 grams I am allowed, then I will most likely have sugar free jello and cool whip.

On the other hand, if it only comes up to say 30 grams of Carb. then I chose a dish of ice cream or Chocolate Pudding with cool whip.

I like to cut my meals a little short so that I can have a fair sized snack in the evening. By cutting my mealtime intake to 40 grams, it allows me approx. 35 grams for a snack at 9:00 PM.

Proper choice here also allows a lot of food to pass your lips. I like an open faced sandwich with cheese, and cotto salami on dark bread. Neither the cheese nor the salami contains any Carbohydrates and the bread only 17 gr. which is very low for the evening snack before bedtime, yet is filling enough to be satisfying.

Here is a discovery I have made about **FAST FOOD.** Several times I have stopped at Burger King for a Whopper or Mac Donalds for their 1/4 pounder with a cup of coffee or diet drink. Almost everytime I have a reaction of low blood sugar (or Hypoglocema) about 3 hours later! Reason? The bun is the only Carbohydrate!

Here again, when I feel the effects such as quivering or slight shaking, flushing or sweating, or numbness in the legs as you might feel when you have over exercised, I immediately test my blood count. I feel these symptoms when my count is 70 to 80 points. Other diabetics may go as low as 60 before feeling these effects.

A banana and one fig cookie takes care of it, but without the test, I may have waited for my evening meal with even greater discomfort or dizziness. While a coma is seldom developed by one on oral medicine, it could reach a point that would make it dangerous to drive, or cause you to fall, or just feeling doopy.

Besides, why suffer the discomfort of upset stomach, shakes, etc. when a little intake of a simple sugar will quickly rectify the condition? **Again, buy a monitor.**

You will still need to have your blood count taken by a lab and consult with your doctor about the results at least every six months.

He undoubtedly will order a full set of tests with your yearly examination which will indicate the condition of your liver, your kidneys, your urine analysis, cholesterol, etc.

One test that most physician require for their diabetic patients is what is called, **GLYCATED HEMOGLOBIN TEST.** The lab technician measures the concentration of hemoglobin molecules, which are found in red blood cells, that have glucose attached to them. This tells what your average blood glucose level was over the past three to four months. low level is 5% in persons without diabetes. 9% is considered high, with 7% as considered good for a diabetic with 6% being excellent. **My last test was 5.4%**

This is believed even more important than the daily readings you take as it gives a long term reading of control rather than the swings experienced during the day caused by food intake or exercise.

Included will be a chart which I drew up for my own use showing values of Carb. - Fat - Protein - and Calories of many of the foods I usually eat in an easy to read form. There will also be a chart which shows Carbohydrates and Calories only. Since I am more concerned with the amount of Carbohydrates consumed than the other factors, I use this chart more frequently.

In the final pages of this book I will show normal meal plans which I frequently consume that are within the confines of a 1500 to 1800 calorie diet or approx. 155 grams of Carbohydrates per day.

Don't expect any exotic recipes! This will be suggestions for everyday, Family type of meals. Meat & Potato meals if you will, (but go easy on the potatoes.)

Chapter 5

WATCHING NUTRITION FACTS

On pages to follow, are shown several nutrition fact charts as they appear on all packaged food products that you will purchase in the grocery store.

The facts that you will be most interested in is the serving size, and number of servings per container - Calories per serving - and **total carbohydrates.**

Do not be misled by the term, "Sugar Free" or "No sugar added" as the label will often show that they contain more Carbohydrates than those containing sugar.

The reason for this is that other forms of starches or carbohydrates must be added to maintain the proper consistancy or taste and while it may be good for the dieting person, it may not necessarily be true for a diabetic.

You will find many examples of foods often touted as great for healthy eating such as rice, potato skins, pasta, etc. are in direct contrast for consumption by diabetics! Some cereals with no sugar added are actually much higher in Carbohydrate content than some sugar sweetened cereals.

Content of Carbohydrates and Calories will vary for the same item, not only in this book, but also on the Nutrition Facts as shown on the purchased item.

Here again, each product does not have the same formula or recipe to produce it as other firms. Pumpernickel Bread, for example, produced by one of the largest bakery firms in the country may have a Carb. rating of 32 grams per slice while most sliced breads contain only 17 grams.   While more sweeteners or syrups may have been used to increase the quality of taste, the larger size of the individual slice also will be a factor.

In chosing cereal, you will find that the original grain used in its production has an effect on the amount of carbohydrates in the product. Cereals made from Oats seems to have the lowest amount of carbohydrates of all the grains used before processing.   Rather than eating 3 meals a day which is customary for most, I usually divide my meals into 4 parts.

Breakfast - - after rising around 7:00 AM
Noon Lunch- - As close as possible to 12:00 noon
(Afternoon Snack - - 2:30 or 3:00)
Dinner - - 5:00 PM to 6:00 PM
Late Evening - - 8:30 to 9:00 PM

For the advantage of simplicity, I estimate 400 calories and 55 grams of Carbohydrates for all meals. Breakfast - Lunch - and Late Evening usually run some what lower, allowing for more at dinner time and also a light afternoon snack around 2:30 or 3:00.

Nutrition Fact Labels

REGULAR GARLIC RANCH DRESSING
NUTRITION FACTS
Serving size 2tbsp
Calories 180
Total Fat 19g
Cholesterol 10mg
Sodium 270mg
TOTAL CARBOHYDRATES 1g
Protein 0g

FATFREE RANCH DRESSING
NUTRITION FACTS
Serving size   2 tbsp
Calories 50
Total Fat 0g
Cholesterol 0mg
TOTAL CARBOHYDRATES 11g
Protein 0g

WHOLE KERNEL CORN (FROZEN)
NUTRITION FACTS
Serving size   1/2 cup
Calories 80
Total Fat 0.5g
Cholesterol 0mg
Sodium 360mg
TOTAL CARBOHYDRATES 18g
Protein 2g

What is best here? Corn or Green Beans?
Corn - 1/2 cup 18g Carb. - Calories 80
Beans- one cup- 4g Carb. - Calories 25

```
GREEN BEANS (FROZEN)
NUTRITION FACTS
Serving size   1cup
Calories  25
Total Fat  0g
Cholesterol  0mg
Sodium  10mg
TOTAL CARBOHYDRATES  4g
Protein  1g
```

Don't overlook the benefits of TV Dinners. Quick to prepare, low Carb. content & cheap too.

```
MEXICAN ENCHILADA TV DINNER
NUTRITION FACTS
Serving size   1 meal
Calories  360
Total Fat  11g
Cholesterol  20mg
Sodium  1390mg
TOTAL CARBOHYDRATES  55g
Protein  10g
```

```
MEAT LOAF TV DINNER
NUTRITION FACTS
Serving size   1meal
Calories  280
Total Fat  16g
Cholesterol  60mg
Sodium  1020 mg
TOTAL CARBOHYDRATES  23g
Protein  12g
```

```
FAMILY SIZED CHINESE STIR-FRY
PACKAGED DINNER (You add meat)
NUTRITION FACTS
Serving size  1 - 1/4 cup
Calories  50
Total Fat  0g
Cholesterol  0mg
Sodium  450mg
TOTAL CARBOHYDRATES  9g
Protein  10g
```

SODA CRACKERS
NUTRITION FACTS
Serving size   5 crackers
Calories 60
Total Fat 1.5g
Cholesterol 0mg
Sodium 150mg
TOTAL CARBOHYDRATES 11g
Protein 1g

VEG. BEEF WITH BARLEY SOUP
NUTRITION FACTS
Serving size 1/2 cup condensed
(Add equal amt. of water)
Calories 80
Total Fat 2g
Cholesterol 15mg
Sodium 920mg
TOTAL CARBOHYDRATES 11g
Protein 5g

CHICKEN NOODLE SOUP
NUTRITION FACTS
Serving size 1/2 cup condensed
(Add equal amt. of water)
Calories 70
Total Fat 2g
Cholesterol 15mg
Sodium 980mg
TOTAL CARBOHYDRATES 9g
Protein 3g

PASTA & RICE-Healthy in most respects
but not the best for diabetics. Too high
Carb. content.

PASTA OR SPAGHETTI
NUTRITION FACTS
Serving size 2 oz. before cooking
Calories 210
Total Fat 1g
Cholesterol 0mg
Sodium 0mg
TOTAL CARBOHYDRATES 42g
Protein 7g

INSTANT RICE
NUTRITION FACTS
Serving size 3/4 cup (prepared)
Calories 160
Total Fat 0g
Cholesterol 0mg
Sodium 5mg
TOTAL CARBOHYDRATES 36g
Protein 4g

SUGAR FREE GELATIN
NUTRITION FACTS
Serving size 1/2 cup (prepared)
Calories 10
Total Fat og
Sodium 80mg
TOTAL CARBOHYDRATES 1g
Protein 1g

SUGAR FREE CHOCOLATE PUDDING
NUTRITION FACTS
Serving size 1/2 cup (prepared)
Calories 90
Total Fat 0g
Cholesterol 0mg
Sodium 110mg
TOTAL CARBOHYDRATES 7g
Protein 1g

COOL WHIP TOPPING
NUTRITION FACTS
Serving size 2 tbsp.
Calories 25
Total Fat 1.5g
Sodium 0mg
TOTAL CARBOHYDRATES 2g
Protein 3g

SUGAR FREE ICE CREAM
NUTRITION FACTS
Serving size 1/2 cup
Calories 90
Total Fat 3g
Cholesterol 10mg
Sodium 60mg
TOTAL CARBOHYDRATES 17g
Protein 3g

RYE CRISP WAFERS
NUTRITION FACTS
Serving size 2 slices
Calories 70
Total Fat 1g
Cholesterol 0mg
Sodium 55mg
TOTAL CARBOHYDRATES 14g
Protein 14g

SUGAR FREE HOT CHOCOLATE
NUTRITION FACTS
Serving size 1 packet or cup
Calories 50
Total Fat 1g
Cholesterol 0mg
Sodium 125mg
TOTAL CARBOHYDRATES 9g

SUGAR FREE PANCAKE SYRUP
NUTITION FACTS
Serving size 1/4 cup
Calories 35
Total Fat 0g
Cholesterol 0mg
Sodium 80mg
TOTAL CARBOHYDRATES 9g
Protein 0g

REGULAR PANCAKE SYRUP
NUTRITION FACTS
Serving size 1/4 cup
Calories 230
Total Fat 0g
Sodium 55mg
TOTAL CARBOHYDRATES 58g
Protein 0g

NOTE: 58 Grams Carb. and 230 Calories.
Compare this with Sugar Free Syrup above.

FROZEN PREPARED WAFFLES
NUTRITION FACTS
Serving size 2 waffles
Calories 190
Total Fat 6g
Cholesterol 0mg
Sodium 530mg
TOTAL CARBOHYDRATES 29G
Protein 4g

```
LOW FAT MILK
NUTRITION FACTS
Serving size  1 cup
Calories  110
Total Fat  2.5g
Cholesterol  10mg
Sodium  125mg
TOTAL CARBOHYDRATES  13g
Protein  8g
```

Always add Carb. content of milk when used to make puddings or put on cereals.

```
REGULAR SOFT DRINKS
NUTRITION FACTS
Serving size  1 can
Calories  180
Total Fat  0g
Sodium  45mg
TOTAL CARBOHYDRATES  48g
Protein  0g
```

A diabetic should not even consider drinking a soft drink other than DIET SOFT DRINKS. With 48 grams in each glass, three in one day would allow no other food consumption that day.

```
DIET SOFT DRINK
NUTRITION FACTS
Total Fat  0g
Sodium  10mg
TOTAL CARBOHYDRATES  0g
Protein  0g
```

FIRST OF ALL, I WANT TO EMPHASIZE THAT I AM NOT ATTEMPTING TO DOWN PLAY THE ADVISE OF YOUR DOCTOR CONCERNING THE TREATMENT OF YOUR PHASE II DIABETES. HIS OPINION COMES FIRST!

What I am trying to convey to you is a method of control plan that has worked very well for me in reducing my glucose blood readings, loss of excess weight, and even reduction in the amount of medication that I have been taking.

Many books are published showing information as to Carbohydrate, Calories, Fat content, and other data to aid persons who wish to maintain a proper diet for their particular needs.

What may be good for an athlete or average person without diabetes may be in direct contrast to that diet which is good for a Phase II Diabetic.

Since this book is geared for those of us that have Phase II Diabetes, I am cutting down on the degree of facts in order to make it more functional and easy to read. Too much included only makes it harder to find the figures that you are looking for as well as being very time consuming.

The charts to follow are simplified to show only Carbohydrate content of certain foods and also the Calories of a normal serving. While Carbohydrate content is of most value to the diabetic, Calories are included so that you can stay within range of the diet prescribed by your Doctor.

It could be possible that you could go overboard in your conservation of Carbohydrates by eating a large amount of meats or cheese that contain little or no Carbohydrates, but this is not a healthy thing to do either. A good balance is essential.

Those of you that have problems with High Blood Pressure, cholesterol, or heart conditions will have to be more cautious than I have been since I do not have any of these other conditions. In this case, you may want to purchase those books that show pertinent facts for each food indicating fat content, salt, protein, etc.

The foods shown in the charts are more or less everyday items that occur in the meals of the average family. Your taste for certain items will determine which ones are best for you that show a low Carbohydrate figure as well as Calories.

I suggest that you take this book to your Doctor and see if he approves of the applications shown for your particular condition before undertaking the diet that has worked so well for me.

What should your desired Glucose levels be?

Confusion is quite understandble as it varies from Patient to Patient. Your age, time of test, results of the Glycated Hemoglobin test as evaluated by your Doctor. As a Phase II diabetic not on insulin, this test should be taken at least every six months. Generally speaking, the goals you set for yourself should be as follows.

> Before Meals   80 to 120mg/dl
> Before Bedtime 100 to 140 mg/dl

Some years ago, a person over 65 with a reading of 140 to 180 after fasting was acceptible. Now this is no longer true. **Don't be shy. Ask your Doctor what your goal should be.**

1500 CALORIE DIET CHARTS

1500 CALORIE DIET
CARBOHYDRATES   155 GR.
PROTEIN   70 GR.
FATS   70 GR.

FOOD EATEN	Carb.	Protein	Fat	Calories
Bacon 3 cooked	0	5		80
Imit. Crab (2 oz)	3			
Meat (3 Oz)	0	21	15	219
Chicken	0	29	1.5	140
Cheese (1oz)	1	7	1	110
Eggs (1)	1	7	4	70
Milk (1 cup)	12	9	25	110
Salami	0	4	6	70
Sausage (3 links)	19	7	19	210
Bratwurst (Johnsoville) (1)	1	14	25	290

BAKERY

	Carb.	Protein	Fat	Calories
Bread (1 slice)	15	2	0	70
Cookie (1)	9	1	5	80
Crackers (5)	11	1	1.5	60
Rye Crisp (2 pcs)	10	2	0	50
Toast(2pcs)	28	3	1	160
Waffles (2sqs)	29	3	2	190
Stuffing	20	3	1	180
Muffin	25	4	1	130
French toast (2)	32	11	8	280

SOUPS

Soup per serving(1/2 cup)	Carb.	Protein	Fat	Calories
Beef w/Barley	11	5	2	80
Chicken & Mushroom	9	3	9	80
Cr. of Mushroom	9	2	7	110
Tomato				

CEREALS

Cheerios	23	3	2	160
Corn Flakes (Bowl)	24	2	0	100
Honey nut	24	3	2.5	170
Oatmeal	18	5	3	190
Wheat & Bran Cereal	47	7	1	200

Item	Carb.	Protein	Fat	Calories
MISC.				
Jelly(1 Tbsp)	13	0	0	50
Margarine(1 Tsp)	0	0	5	45
SF Syrup 1/4 cup	9	0	0	35
Reg. Syrup (1/4 cup)	58	0	0	230

DESSERTS

Choc. Pudding (SF)	4	1	2.5	90
Cool Whip (2 Tbsp)	2	0	1.5	25
Cookie (1)	9	1	5	80
Ice Cream (SF 1/2 cup)	17	4	7	140
Ice Cream Reg.(1/2 cup)	19	2	2	130
Ice Cream Choc bar	10	2	5	10

FRUITS & VEGATABLES

Banana (one)	10	0	0	40
Corn(2/3 cup)	18	3	1	80
Pasta (3/4 cup)	40	9	2	210
Potato (1 small)	30	2	0	210
Squash 1/3 cup	8	1	0	30
Vegetables (1/2 cup)	5	2	0	25
Carrots (3 oz.)	9	1	0	44
Spinach (1/3 cup)	2	2	0	20

Winton N. Petersen

MISC.

Hash	19	19	24	350
Honey Baked Beans 1/2cp	29	—	1	140
Orange Juice 1 cup	29	1	0	120
Peanut Butter	7	7	16	190
Ranch Dressing (2 tbsp)	1	0	19	180
Stirfry (Chic or beef)	20	6	5	310
Tuna Helper	33	6	4	310
Pasta Roni (cup prepared)	45	9	6	420

JUNK FOOD

Potato Chips (19)	14	2	10	150
Popcorn (5 cups)	24	4	1	100
Reg. Coke(8oz)	25	0	0	100
Diet Drinks	0	0	0	0
S.F. Hot Choc.	8	3	2.5	70

FAST FOODS

MCDONALD'S

ITEM	CARB.	FAT GRAMS	PROTEIN	CALORIES
Plain Breakfast Biscuit	32	31	5	290
With Meat	33	23	11	470
Pancakes & syrup (3)	100	16	9	570
Big Mac	45	31	26	560
Quarter Pounder	37	21	23	420
Chicken McNuggets (6)	15	17	18	290
French Fries (Small)	26	10	3	210
Apple Pie	34	13	3	260
Shake (small)	60	9	11	360
Sundae, Hot Fudge	52	12	8	340
Garden Salad	7	0	2	35
Ranch Dressing	10	21	1	230

BURGER KING

Crossan'wich				
Bacon, egg & cheese	18	24	15	350
Hash Browns	25	12	2	220
Whopper	45	39	27	630
Whopper Junior	29	24	21	410
Chicken Sandwich	54	43	26	700
BK-Big Fish Sandwich	59	43	25	720
Chicken Tenders (6)	14	12	16	250

ARBY'S

Jr. Roast Beef Sandwich	35	14	17	324
Reg. Roast Beef Sand.	33	19	23	388
Breaded Chicken Fillet	46	28	28	536
French Dip	40	22	30	475
Curley Fries	38	15	4	300
Turnovers	46	13	4	320
cheese Cake	23	23	5	320

The forms shown on the previous pages display not only the Carbohydrate and Calorie values of certain foods, but also values of Fat content and Protein.

This is for the use of those persons that have other physical ailments that require that they watch these items as well.

For persons with heart and circulation problems, Nutritional Facts concerning Sodium, Cholesterol, Saturated Fats, Dietary Fiber, etc. can be found on the label of Nutritional Facts that is a part of packaging of all commercially produced food purchased in the Grocery Store.

The Fast Food Chart showing values of Carbohydrates, Fat, Protein, and Calories is for quick reference when you are away from home. While only a few of the Fast Food Outlets are displayed here, it can be a guide for similar products sold at competing restaurants.

The following charts show only the carbohydrate contents in grams for quick reference for those of us who are most concerned with out Blood Sugar Control.

CARBOHYDRATE COUNTS
FAST FOODS

MCDONALD'S	Carbohydrates in Grams
Biscuits	
plain.......	32
Sausage, egg	33
Burrito.....	23
Eggs, scrambled...	1.0
Hash Browns...	14
Hotcakes....	53
Hotcakes, syrup, & Margarine....	100
Sausage, (alone)	0
MUFFINS	
Egg McMuffin...	27
English....	25
Sausage Mcmuffin..	26
with egg...	27
Apple Bran muffin...	61
Apple Danish...	51
Cinnamon Roll..	47

SANDWICHES	CARBOHYDRATES IN GRAMS
Big Mac........	*45*
Cheeseburger...........	*35*
Crispy Chicken Deluxe...	*43*
Fish Filet Deluxe.........	*54*
Hamburger..........	*34*
Quarter Pounder......	*37*
with Cheese..........	*38*

CHICKEN MCNUGGETS:

6 piece........	*15*
9 piece.......	*23*
Sauces (10 to 12 grams each)	

FRENCH FRIES;

Small....................	*26*
Large...................	*57*
Supersized..........	*68*

SALADS....................(ALL)	*7*

Dressings:

Caesar................	*7*
Ranch................	*10*
Red French, (Reduced Cal.)	*23*

DESSERTS & SHAKES

Baked Apple Pie......	*34*
Choc. Chip Cookie....	*22*
Ice Cream Cone.......	*23*
Choc. Shake.....(small)	*60*
Vanilla Shake ...(small)	*59*
Sundae, Hot Caramel.......	*61*

Sundae, Hot Fudge...........	*52*
Sundae, Strawberry..........	*50*
Sundae, Nuts..................	*2*

BURGER KING

BREAKFAST

Biscuit, bacon, egg, cheese.......	*39*
Biscuit with sausage...............	*41*
Croissan'wich, sausage, egg, cheese....	*25*
French Toast sticks.........	*60*
Hash browns...............	*25*
Jellies......................(1 pck.)	*7*

SANDWICHES:

BK big fish................	*56*
BK Broiler Chicken.........	*41*
Cheeseburger, Reg, double, or w/bacon...	*28*
Chicken Sandwich....	*54*
Double Whopper, Reg......	*45*
with cheese.................	*46*
Hamburger......................	*28*
Whopper.........................	*45*
with cheese................	*46*
Whopper Jr...................	*29*

Chicken Tenders, 8 pcs.....	*19*
Sauces:	
A.M. Express............	*21*
barbecue.................	*9*
Bullseye...............	*5*
Honey...................	*23*
ranch....................	*2*
Sweet & Sour........	*11*
FRIES - Regular.........	*43*
Onion Rings..............	*41*
Salads, no dressing........	*7*

Salad Dressings:	***CARBOHYDRATES IN GRAMS***
Blue Cheese...........	*1*
French..................	*11*
Italian, light...........	*3*
Ranch...................	*2*
Thousand Island......	*7*
SHAKES: (Medium)	
Chocolate...............	*54*
Chocolate with syrup...	*84*
Strawberry with syrup..	*83*
Vanilla.......................	*53*
Dutch Apple Pie.............	*39*

ARBY'S

BREAKFAST:

Bacon, 2 strips...	**0**
Biscuit, plain..........	**34**
Blueberry Muffin.....	**35**
Cinnamon-nut Danish.....	**60**
Croissant, plain..............	**25**
Egg portion....................	**5**
French Toastix, 6 pieces....	**52**

CARBOHYDRATES IN GRAMS

Ham or Sausage................	**0**
Table Syrup......................	**25**

SANDWICHES ....
Chicken:

Breaded Fillet	**46**
Cordon Bleau................	**46**
Grilled, BBQ...............	**47**
Grilled, DeLuxe.....	**41**
Fish Fillet.........................	**50**
Ham & Cheese..................	**34**

ROAST BEEF SANDWICHES;

Arby's Melt with Chedder...	**36**
Arby " Q"....	**48**
Bacon, Chedder Deluxe...	**38**
Beef & Chedder..............	**40**

Giant...........................   *43*

Junior..........................   *35*

Regular........................   *33*

Super...........................   *50*

SUB-ROLL:
    French Dip.....................   *40*

    Hot Ham & Swiss...........   *43*

    Italian Sub.....................   *46*

    Philly Beef & Swiss.......   *48*

    Roast Beef Sub..............   *44*

    Triple Cheese Melt.......   *46*

    Turkey Sub.................   *47*
                                         12

Soups:
    Boston Clam Chowder....   *18*

    Cream of Broccoli...........   *15*

    Cheese...........................   *20*

    Chicken Noodle............   *11*

    Chili..........................   *17*

    Potato w/ bacon........   *23*

    Vegatable..................   *10*

CARBOHYDRATES IN GRAMS

POTATOES - BAKED
　　　Plain.........　　　　　　　　　　　　　　82

　　　Margarine & sour Cream.......　　　　　85

　　　Broccoli 'n Chedder..............　　　　89

Curly Fries.................　　　　　　　　38

　　　With Chedder.......　　　　　　　　　　40

French Fries..............　　　　　　　　30

Sauces:
　　　Arby's Sauce.........　　　　　　　　　4

　　　Barbecue Sauce...　　　　　　　　　　1

　　　Au Jus ....　　　　　　　　　7

　　　Blue Cheese.........　　　　　　　　　2

　　　Buttermilk ranch, reduced Calories　　12

　　　Honey French　　　　　　　　　　　18

　　　HORSEY SAUCE...........　　　　　2

DESSERTS:
　　　Apple Turnover...........　　　　　　48

　　　Cheesecake.................　　　　　　23

CARBOHYDRATES IN GRAMS

Polor Swirl:
　　　Butterfinger...............　　　　　　62

　　　Heath.......................　　　　　　76

　　　Oreo.........................　　　　　66

Snickers.................... 73

Peanut Butter Cup......... 61

SHAKES:
Chocolate..................... 76

Jamocha..................... 62

Vanilla...................... 50

WENDY'S
Sandwiches:

Bacon Cheeseburger, Jr.............. 34

Big Bacon Classic...................... 46

Cheeseburger, Jr...................... 34

Cheeseburger Deluxe, Jr......... 36

Chicken, Breaded.................. 44

Chicken, Grilled..................... 35

Chciken, Spicy..................... 43

Chicken, Club...................... 44

CARBOHYDRATES IN GRAMS

Hamburger, single, Plain.... 31

Hamburger, single, w/everything... 37

Hamburger, Jr. 35

Chicken Nuggets, 5 pieces..... 7

Chilli -

small,........................ 21

Large........................	*32*
Baked Potato:	
Plain........................	*71*
Bacon & Cheese...........	*78*
Broccoli & Cheese.......	*80*
Cheese........................	*78*
Chili and Cheese.........	*83*
Sour Cream & Chive...	*74*
Fries:	
Small...........................	*33*
Medium........................	*47*
Biggie..........................	*58*
Salads: (No Dressing)..............	*10*
Taco Salad..........................	*53*
Soft Bread Stick................	*24*
Desserts:	
Choc. Chip Cookie (1) ...	*38*
Frosty, small..................	*57*
Frosty, Medium............	*76*
Frosty, Large.................	*95*

Following are selected items from Denny's Restaurant chain that is a fair representation of menus of any number of other eating establishments. The meals shown have been pulled out to illustrate what is available for the average person that has Phase II diabetes and and also indicates that there are a number of items available that are actually within the limits of the required diet.

Even though you may frequent another food location, by referring to this information, you can chose wisely what you should be eating for health and yet select what is pleasing to your taste.

Of course their entire menu is not shown, but most items are those that are acceptable to one's diet, or , in some cases, those that definately are out of bounds.

DENNY'S RESTAURANT

Breakfast Items

All American Slam.................	*24*
Belgian Waffle, plain............	*23*
Belgian Waffle Supreme, no meat..	*50*
Chicken fried steak and eggs............	*31*
French Slam.......................	*58*
French Toast, plain, 2 pcs...............	*51*
Ham & Cheddar Omelette.................	*24*
Original Grand Slam, no syrup or butter	*65*
Pancakes, plain, (3).......................	*95*
Senior Starter, no meats................	*36*
Senior Belgian Waffle Slam, no syrup	*12*
Senior Omlette.............................	*27*
Sugar Free syrup................	*6*
Reg. Syrup..........................	*36*
Bacon.................4 strips....	*1*
Egg, one.............................	*1*
Ham............3 oz.................	*2*
Sausage......4 links............	*0*

Grits, 4 oz......................	*18*
Hash browns.......................	*20*
Bagel, one whole..................	*46*
Orange juice, 10 oz...............	*31*
Toast, dry, 1 slice.................	*17*

Senior Meals:

Battered Cod, without potato or rice..	*7*
Chicken Fried Steak...........................	*29*
Grilled Chicken Breast......................	*16*
Liver, bacon & onions......................	*20*
Pork Chop...	*0*
Pot Roast..	*6*
Turkey, and stuffing.........................	*61*

(Add to this choice of soup or salad & 2 vegetables)
Entrees:

Battered cod with tartar sauce........	*48*
Chicken fried steak.........................	*14*
Chicken strip with honey-mustard dressing.	*55*
Prime Rib (8 oz) au jus & horseradish......	*8*
Grilled Alaskan Salmon..........................	*1*
Grilled Breast of Chicken.......................	*0*
Liver,Bacon & Onions............................	*13*
Pork Chop Dinner................................	*0*
Porterhouse Steak...............................	*0*
Roast Turkey & Dressing,......................	*63*
Steak & Shrimp.....................................	*31*
Shrimp...	*49*
T Bone Steak.......................................	*0*

(Add to this choice of salad, soup, or fruit, choice of potato or rice pilaf, and choice of vegetable.)

SEE NEXT PAGE FOR CHOICES

Broccoli in butter sauce...............	*7*
Carrots in honey glaze..................	*12*
Corn in butter sauce....................	*19*
Corn bread stuffing.....................	*20*
French fries...............................	*35*
Green Beans with bacon............	*6*
Green Peas in butter sauce.......	*14*
Baked Potato..............................	*43*

Mashed Potato..............................	*21*
Rice pilaf.......................................	*21*
Sliced Tomato (3)........................	*3*

Pies:

Apple...	*59*
Apple with equal........................	*43*
Cheesecake pie............................	*48*
Choc. Pecan................................	*107*
Coconut Cream...........................	*58*
Key Lime....................................	*71*
Lemon Meringue.....................	*71*
Pecan.......................................	*81*

When it comes to desserts, best to split one with your partner or skip them entirely after a full meal.

THE GLYCEMIC INDEX

The following chart showing the glycemic index of certain foods is for your information should you wish to learn more about it and also the effects in has in your diet as a Diabetic.

All carbohydrates such as fructose found in most fruits, sucrose, common sugar, starch, etc. are broken down into glucose. A higher glycemic index means that more carbohydrates are stored away as fatty tissue rather than being burned up.

Having too many high glycemic foods in our diet is one of the reasons that the average American is getting fatter or has a weight problem.

High glycemic foods have also been shown to increase appetite and craving for food.

For the Diabetic, it is suggested that they eat as many as possible, the foods that are low glycemic foods, preferably from 55 to 70 on a white bread scale of 100. Since high glycemic foods have a tendency to cause production of insulin, (while you may think this is desirable), it may cause a sudden swing to hypoglycemic or low blood sugar which could, in the case of insulin dependent Diabetics, even result in a coma.

This is a highly complicated subject and before taking any action, I suggest you confer with your Doctor.

Value Food

Value	Food
152	Maltose
138	Glucose
134	Cooked Parsnips
132	Puffed Rice
131	Lucozade
128	Potato, russet, baked
126	Honey
121	Rice, instant, boiled 6 min.
118	Potato, instant
117	Cooked Carrots

Value Food

Value	Food
115	Cornflakes
109	Wheatabix
109	Broad beans (Fava beans)
103	Millet

100	Potato, mashed
100	Tortilla, corn
100	Bread, wheat, whole meal
100	Bread, wheat, white
99	Rutabaga (swede)
99	Corn Chips
97	Shredded Wheat
96	Muesli
95	Cookies, ryvita
95	Bread, rye, crispbread
94	Mars bar
91	Cookies, plain crackers
91	Apricots, canned
89	Sucrose
89	Bread, rye, whole meal
88	Raisins
88	Beetroot
87	Porridge, oats
84	Banana
82	Cookies, digestive
81	Rice, brown
81	Pastry
80	Sweet corn
80	Potato, new, boiled

Value	Food
80	Cookies, rich, tea
79	Rice, polished, boiled 15 min.
79	Fruit Cocktail
78	Cookies, Oatmeal
77	Potato Chips
74	Yams
74	Peaches, canned
74	Buckwheat
74	All bran
70	Potato, sweet
69	Grapefruit
68	Bread, rye, pumpernickel
66	Pineapple juice
65	Rice, boiled 25 min.
65	Rice, instant, boiled 1 min.
65	Green peas, marrowfat
65	Green beans, frozen
63	Wheat kernels

63	Sponge cake
63	Pears, canned
62	Grapes
61	Spaghetti, white, boiled 15 min.
60	Baked beans, canned
59	Orange
58	Rice, pollished, boiled 5 min.
58	Pears
57	Haricot (white) beans
54	Brown beans
53	Apple
52	Yogurt
52	Tomato soup
52	Ice Cream
52	Fish fingers
50	Lima beans
50	Green peas, dried

Value	Food
49	Whole milk
49	Chick peas (garbanzo)
48	2% milk
47	Rye kernels
46	Skim milk
46	Butter beans
46	Blackeyed peas
46	Apricots, dried
45	Spaghetti,white, boiled 5 min.
45	Kidney beans
43	Black beans
40	Peaches
39	Sausages
38	Pasta, protein enriched
37	Red lentils
34	Plum
31	Fructose
67	Orange juice
31	Barley, pearled
22	Soy beans, canned
20	Soy beans, dried
15	Peanuts
12	Bengal gram dal
10	Nopal (Prickly pear)

CARBOHYDRATE – CALORIE DIET

1500 CALORIE DIET
DAILY ALLOWANCE OF CARBOHYDRATES — 155 GRAMS

BEVERAGES

ITEM	SERVING SIZE	CARB.	CALORIES
Milk (1%)	1 cup	13 grams	110
Sugar Free Hot Chocolate	1 packet	9 grams	50
Diet Soft Drinks	8 oz. glass	0 grams	0
Sugar Sweetened Orange Soda	12 oz. can	48 grams	180
Orange Juice	1 Cup	29 grams	120
Grapefruit Juice	1 Cup	24 grams	100
Cranberry Juice Cocktail	8 oz. glass	35 grams	145
Cranapple Juice	8 oz. glass	40 grams	175

BREADS

ITEM	SERVING SIZE	CARB.	CALORIES
100% whole Wheat Bread	1 Slice	10 grams	50
Pecan Breakfast Bread	1 Slice	14 grams	80
Seeded Rye Bread	1 Slice	14 grams	70
Frozen Waffles	1 waffles	29 grams	190
White Bread	1 Slice	11 grams	50
Rye Crisp	2 Slices	14 grams	70

Soda Crackers   5 Crackers   11 grams   60
Bagel   one   44 grams   210

CEREALS

ITEM	SERVING SIZE	CARB.	CALORIES
Grape Nuts	1/2 cup	47 grams	200
Honey Bunch of Nuts	3/4 cup	24 grams	130
Cap't Crunch	3/4 cup	23 grams	110
Cheerios	1 cup	22 grams	110
Oatmeal (Cooked)	1 cup	27 grams	150
2% Milk	1/2 cup	6 1/2 grams	150

Milk is shown here as most cereals are eaten with milk added. When consumed with milk, the Carb. and Calorie figures should be added to the cereal contents.

Nutritional value of the above should not be determined solely on the above figures, as these figures pertain to use of these products from the diabetic viewpoint.

Cereals made from Oats appear to have the lowest amount of Carbohydrates present.

DESSERTS AND FRUITS

ITEM	SERVING SIZE	CARB.	CALORIES
Sugar Free Jello	1/2 cup	1 gram	10
Regular Jello	1/2 cup	19 grams	80
Sugar Free Cook & Serve Choc. Pudding	1/2 cup	7 grams	90
Sugar Free Ice Cream	1/2 cup	13 grams	90
Regular-Choc. Almond Ice Cream	1/2 cup	17 grams	170
Cool Whip Topping	2 Tablespoons	2 grams	25
Pears (Canned) Lite	1/2 cup	15 grams	60
Oranges	one	17 grams	75
Banana	one	10 grams	40
Apple	one	21 grams	75

FAST FOODS

ITEM	SERVING SIZE	CARB.	CALORIES

MC DONALD'S

BREAKFST ITEMS

ITEM	SERVING SIZE	CARB.	CALORIES
Breakfast Biscuit (plain)	one	32 grams	290
Breakfast Biscuit w/sausage	one	33 grams	470
Pancakes w/syrup	three	100 grams	570

MEALTIME ITEMS

ITEM	SERVING SIZE	CARB.	CALORIES
Big Mac	one	45 grams	560
Qtr Pounder	one	37 grams	420
Chicken Mcnuggets	six	15 grams	290
French Fries	small	26 grams	210
Apple pie	one	34 grams	260
Ice Cream Shake	small	60 grams	360
Sundae (Choc.)	one	52 grams	340
Garden Salad	one	7 grams	35
Ranch Dressing	one pkt	10 grams	230

ITEM	SERVING SIZE	CARB.	CALORIES
BURGER KING			
Croissan'wich sausage & egg	one	25 grams	530
Hashbrowns	one pc.	25 grams	220
Whopper	one	45 grams	630
Chicken Sand.	one	54 grams	700
Onion Rings	small	41 grams	310
ARBY'S			
Curly fries	Regular	38 grams	300
Roast Beef Sand.	Regular	33 grams	388
Fish Sand.	one	50 grams	529
Horsey Sauce	one Tblsp.	2 grams	60
Baked Potato with sour cream	one	85 grams	578
Cheese Cake	one slice	23 grams	320

ITEM	SERVING SIZE	CARB.	CALORIES

WENDY'S

ITEM	SERVING SIZE	CARB.	CALORIES
Jr. Bacon/Cheese burger	one	34 grams	380
Hamburger, plain	one	31 grams	360
Chilli	8 oz.	21 grams	227
Baked Potato Bacon & Cheese	one small	78 grams	380

MEATS AND CHEESE

ITEM	SERVING SIZE	CARB.	CALORIES
Frozen Sand. Steakettes	2 oz. each	0 grams	180
Cotto Salami	1 slice	0 grams	70
Cheese (Cheddar)	1 oz.	0 grams	120
Pork Chop	1 med.	0 grams	225
Beef	3 oz.	0 grams	210

SOUPS
IND. MICROWAVE DINNER CUPS

ITEM	SERVING SIZE	CARB.	CALORIES
MICRO-CUPS			
Rice, Beef, Veg.	1 cup	38 grams	250
Beef Stew	1 cup	17 grams	170
Pasta & Chicken	1 cup	22 grams	150
Chicken & Dumpling	1 cup	21 grams	140
Scalloped Potatoes and Ham	1 cup	20 grams	240

ITEM	SERVING SIZE	CARB.	CALORIES
SOUPS (one can of soup contains 2 1/2 servings)			
Chicken Noodle	1/2 cup	9 grams	70
Beef stock Veg.	1/2 cup	16 grams	80
Beef, Veg. & Barley	1/2 cup	`11 grams	80

PASTA & NOODLES

Vermicelli Spaghetti	1 cup cooked	42 grams	210
Red Spaghetti Sauce	1/2 cup	23 grams	140
Clam Sauce	1/2 cup	5 grams	140
Alfredo Sauce	1/4 cup	3 grams	120
Chinese Noodles	1/2 cup	19 grams	140

SNACK FOODS

ITEM	SERVING SIZE	CARB.	CALORIES
Bugles	1 1/3 cup	18 grams	160
Flavored Snack Mix	1/2 cup	18 grams	170
Peanuts, dry roast	1/4 cup	7 grams	200
Corn Cheese puffs	1 oz.	17 grams	150

VEGETABLES

ITEM	SERVING SIZE	CARB.	CALORIES
Cauliflower-	1 cup	5 grams	30
Broccoli	3/4 cup	4 grams	25
Chopped Spinach	1/3 cup	2 grams	20
French Cut Beans	1 cup	4 grams	25
Green Peas	2/3 cup	12 grams	70
Potato	1 Med. baked	51 grams	125
Potato	1/2 cup mashed	19 grams	180
Squash	1/3 cup	8 grams	30
Tomatoes (canned)	1/2 cup	4 grams	25
Whole Kernel Corn	1/2 cup	18 grams	80
Rice (Cooked)	3/4 cup	36 grams	160

SPREADS AND DRESSINGS

ITEM	SERVING SIZE	CARB.	CALORIES
Stick Margarine	1 tbsp.	0 grams	70
Soft Spread Margarine	1 tbsp.	0 grams	90
Orange Marmalade	1 tbsp.	13 grams	50
Peanut butter	2 tbsp.	7 grams	190
Fat Free Ranch Dressing	2 tbsp.	11 grams	50
Regular Ranch Dressing	2 tbsp.	1 gram	180
Regular Classic Caesar	2 tbsp.	2 grams	100
Regular Tangy Tomato Bacon	2 tbsp.	8 grams	130
Oil and Vinegar	2 tbsp.	0 grams	100
Mayonnaise	1 Tbsp.	2 grams	70

DAILY MEAL MENUS

BREAKFAST	CARB.	CALORIES
French Toast	32	280
2 pcs bacon	0	80
1/2 cup orange juice	15	50
Coffee	0	0
Total Carbohydrates - - 47		
Total Calories - - - - - - - 410		
1 cup oatmeal	27	15
1/2 cup milk	6.5	150
1 PC. toast	11	50
jelly (1 Tbsp.)	13	50
1/2 cup orange juice		
Total Carbohydrates - - 57 1/2		
Total Calories - - - - - - 265		
3 pancakes	45	285
1/4 cup sugar free syrup	9	35
3 pcs. bacon	0	80
coffee	0	0
Total Carbohydrates - - 54		
Total Calories - - - - - - 400		
2 pcs. toast	28	160
2 fried eggs	2	140
1 tbsp. margarine	0	45
Coffee	0	0
Total Carbohydrates - - 30		
Total Calories - - - - - - 345		
2 pcs. white toast	28	160
1 sectioned orange	17	75
1 tablespoon marg.	0	45
2 pkts nutrisweet &		
cinnamon (on toast)	0	0
Total Carbohydrates - -45		
Total Calories - - - - - 280		

1 Burger King Sausage & egg		
Croissan'wich	25	350
Coffee	0	0

Total Carbohydrates - - 25
Total Calories - - - - - - 350

3 pcs. lean bacon	0	70
2 egg Omelette	2	140
1 oz. shredded Cheese	1	90
1 pc. dark toast	12	70

Total Carbohydrates - - 15
Total Calories - - - - - - 460

DINNER	CARB.	CALORIES
3 oz. hamburger patty	0	219
1/2 small potato	15	63
Garden Salad	7	35
2 tbsp. Garlic Ranch dressing	1	180
1/2 cup jello (S.F.)	1	10
2 tbsp. cool whip	2	25

Carbohydrates - - 26
Calories - - - - - - 532

One Med. Pork Chop	0	220
2/3 cup squash	16	60
2 tbsp. Margarine	0	90
1/2 cup stove top dressing	20	180
1/2 cup ice cream	19	130

Carbohydrates - - 61
Calories - - - - - - - 680

One 3 oz. chicken breast	0	140
1/2 cup instant potatoes	6	170
1 cup French cut beans	4	25
1/2 cup S.F. choc. pudding	4	90
2 tbsp. cool whip	2	25

Carbohydrates - - 14
Calories - - - - - - 450

DINNER	CARB.	CALORIES
One 3 oz. Beef Steak	0	219
Garden Salad	7	35
2 tbsp. Reg. dressing	1	180
1/4 cup cubed, grilled potato	15	105
1/2 cup Tapioca Pudding (S.F.)	5	20
2 tbsp. cool whip	5	20

Carbohydrates - - 33
Calories - - - - - - 584

	CARB.	CALORIES
Chicken stirfry	20	310
1/2 cup rice (cooked)	36	160
Iced tea	0	0
S.F. Jello	1	10
2 tbsp. cool whip	2	25
1/2 banana in jello	5	20

Carbohydrates - - 64
Calories - - - - - - 525

S.F. - - - Sugar Free (or with Nutrisweet or similar sweetener)

Tbsp. - - Tablespoon

Caution: 2 oz. of Potato skins contain 16 grams of. Carbohydrates

COLD PLATE

	CARB.	CALORIES
3 oz. cold cuts (Beef, Salami, liverwurst),	0	210
3 oz. Grilled Chicken breast	0	140
1 deviled egg	3	170
6 oz. cole slaw	10	20

Carbohydrates - - 13
Calories - - - - - - 540

DINNERS	CARB.	CALORIES
3 oz. Hamburger Patty	0	219
3/4 cup cut Broccoli	4	25
1/2 sliced tomato	3	13
1/2 cup Cottage Cheese	4	110
1/3 cup squash	8	30
1 tbsp. Margarine	0	90
2 oz. raw onions	5	15

1/2 cup S.F. Choc. pudding (with 2 tbsp. cool whip)	6	115
Carbohydrates - - 30		
Calories - - - - - - 617		

One Grilled Bratwurst	1	290
3 egg omlet (onions & peppers to suit)	2	210
2 oz cheese (in omlet)	2	180
Water, Coffee or Tea	0	0
Carbohydrates - - 5		
Calories - - - - - - 680		

Roast turkey leg 4 oz.	0	175
1/2 cup Instant Potato	17	90
3/4 cup cut broccoli	4	25
1/3 cup squash	8	30
1/2 cup Ice Cream	17	140
Carbohydrates - - 56		
Calories - - - - - 460		

DINNERS	CARB.	CALORIES
TV DINNERS		
(Quick, easy, and supplement with added side dishes)		
Yankee Pot Roast	20	230
Garden Salad	7	90
Bacon, Tom. Dressing	8	130
1/2 cup Ice Cream (Carmel, Vanilla Flavor)	13	140
Carbohydrates - - 52		
Calories - - - - - - - 590		

Chicken Fettuccine	37	420
Garden Salad	7	90
Ranch Dressing	1	190
S.F. Jello w/Cool whip	2	735
Carbohydrates - - 47		
Calories - - - - - - 735		

Pasta w/Sausage		
& Peppers	46	423
1/2 sliced tomato	3	13
1/2 cup cottage cheese	4	110

Carbohydrates - - 46
Calories - - - - - - 423

3 oz. Roast Pork	0	210
3 oz. Carrots	9	44
1/2 cup mashed potato	30	210
1 cup Cauliflower	5	30

Carbohydrates - - 44
Calories - - - - - 494

TV DINNERS (Cont'd)

DINNERS	CARB. (grams)	CALORIES
Beef, Enchilada,Tamale	56	380
Garden Salad	7	90
Caesar Dressing	2	100

Carbohydrates - - 65
Calories - - - - - - 570

Country Inn Roast Turkey	28	250
Garden Salad	7	90
2 tbsp. Oil & Vinegar	0	100
2 fig newton cookies	20	100
Iced Tea	0	0

Carbohydrates - - 55
Calories - - - - - - -540

Roasted Chicken	25	230
Cottage Cheese (1/2 cup)	4	110
1 slice Pinapple	8	75
1/2 cup ice cream S.F.	13	140

Carbohydrates - - 50
Calories- - - - - - - 355

LUNCHES	CARB.	CALORIES
Sandwich		
on Rye Bread	28	140
Cotto Salami (1 slice)	0	70
Cheese (2oz)	2	180
S.F. Jello w/cool whip	2	35
Coffee, tea, or diet drink	0	0
Carbohydrates - - 32		
Calories - - - - - - 425		

Beef Stew Micro-cup	17	170
5 soda crackers	11	60
1/2 cup S.F. Choc. Pudding	4	90
2 tbsp. cool whip	2	25
Carbohydrates - - 34		
Calories - - - - - - 345		

Grilled Cheese Sandwich		
2 slices white bread	22	100
1 tbsp. margarine	0	90
2 oz. cheese	2	180
1/2 cup Choc. Almond		
Ice cream	17	170
Carbohydrates - - 41		
Calories - - - - - - - 540		

(Milk products contain lactose-a form of sugar)

LUNCHES	CARB.	CALORIES
1-1/4 cup beef barley		
soup (1/2 can)	14	100
5 soda crackers	11	60
Iced Tea	0	0
1/2 cup S.F. Choc. pudding	4	90
2 tbsp. cool whip	2	25
Carbohydrates- - 31		
Calories- - - - - - 275		

Sandwich

Chicken breast (microwave)	0	140
2 slices white bread	22	100
1 tbsp. mayonnaise	2	90
lettuce leaf	0	0
Diet Drink	0	0
1/2 cup lite pears	7.5	60

      Carbohydrates - -31.5
      Calories - - - - - - 390

(Use Nutrisweet or some other artificial sweetener to improve taste of reduced sugar items such as lite pears or iced tea.)

LUNCH	CARB.	CALORIES
2 Slices Whole Wheat Bread	20	100
1 slice of Ham	1	30
2 pcs. swiss proc. cheese	2	120
1 tbsp. Salad Dressing	2	70
(Make into Sandwich)		
1/2 cup jello w/2 tbsp. cool		
whip & 1/2 Banana	8	55

      Carbohydrates - -33
      Calories - - - - - - 375

(Leftovers)

1/2 cup zucchini	3.5	50
3/4 cup chopped broccoli	4	25
2 Wieners	4	200
1/2 cup Ice Cream	13	130

      Carbohydrates - -24.5
      Calories - - - - - - 405

SNACKS	CARB.	CALORIES
Hot Chocolate - 1 pkt. S.F.	9	50
1 slice white bread	11	50
1 tbsp. Margarine	0	45
Carbohydrates - -20		
Calories - - - - - - 145		
1 slice luncheon meat	0	70
1 oz. cheese	1	110
1/2 cup Jello w/cool whip	2	35
1 cup tea	0	0
Carbohydrates - - 3		
Calories - - - - - - 215		
2 pcs Rye Crisp	10	50
1 slice cotto Salami	0	70
1 oz. Cheese	1	90
Diet soft Drink	0	0
Carbohydrates - - 11		
Calories - - - - - - - 210		
2 oz. Imit. Crabmeat	3	65
1 tbsp. margarine	0	45
Carbohydrates - -3		
Calories - - - - - - 110		
1 Banana	10	40
2 tbsp. cool whip	2	25
Carbohydrates - - 12		
Calories - - - - - - 65		
2 pcs. rye crisp	10	50
2 tbsp. Marg.	0	90
1 oz. Cheese	1	110
Carbohydrates - - 11		
Calories - - - - - - 250		

One-2 oz. beef steakette	0	180
1 slice W. Wheat Bread	10	50
1 tbsp. margarine	0	45

Carbohydrates - - 10
Calories - - - - - — 275

1/2 cup unsweetened		
Applesauce	15	50
2 Tbsp. Cool Whip	2	25
2 pkts Nutrisweet	0	0
Cinnamon to suit	0	0

Carbohydrates - - 17
Calories - - - - - - 75

EXERCISE
AND CALORIES EXPENDED

Activity	Number of Calories expended in 30 minutes
Walking **(4 miles per hr.)**	135
Jogging **(5 miles per hr.)**	240
Bicycling **(10 miles per hr.)**	200
Swimming	200
High Intensity Aerobics	240
Golf **(No Golf Cart)**	150

GOOD FATS - BAD FATS

While this book stresses the counting of Carbohydrates, you may wish to know just what **Fats** are good for you and those that you should avoid. This is especially true if you already have high cholesterol, high blood pressure, or other heart problems.

The following lists are given for your information:

Saturated or Bad Fats - Try not to use these:

Butter	Lard	Chocolate
Meat fat	Cream Cheese	Bacon
Sour Cream	Solid Shortening	Coconut oil
Palm Oil		

Polyunsaturated Fats - Not good - Not all bad:

Corn Oil	Soybean Oil	Cottonseed Oil
Mayonnaise	Sunflower Oil	Safflower Oil
Salad Dressing	Margarine	

Monounsaturated Fats - The Good Guys

Olive Oil	Canola Oil	Avocados
Peanut Butter	Nuts	

SOME TIPS FROM EXPERIENCE

As we all learned from your school days or college days, practical experience is not always the same as what you learned from the books. Practical experience is the proof of knowledge.

Following are some suggestions to make your diet easier, more enjoyable and possibly not so awful as it might be if you had to find out by hit and miss what is best for you.

1. **Check Nutrition Facts on the package** of the food that you buy, especially for <u>Total Carbohydrates</u>.

2. **Use Sugar Free products.** Use only those that are less in Carbohydrates content than regular items. (Example: Sugar free Jello, Sugar Free Choc. Pudding, Sugar Free Hot Chocolate, etc.) Be aware that Sugar Free does not necessarily reduce Carbohydrate content. Again, check labels of both products.

3. **Use artificial sweeteners where you formerly used sugar.** This can be items you are cooking, such as Tapioca Pudding.

4. **Check your Blood Sugar.** If possible, check your blood sugar if you begin to feel light-headed, sweaty, shaky on the inside, or just don't feel good. It may or may not be low blood sugar but if it is below normal, eat half a banana, a few raisins, or drink a little orange juice.

5. **Do not skip meals, especially breakfast.** You have been away from food for several hours and need some Carbohydrates to replace those used during your sleeping hours.

6. **Always carry some form of simple sugar.** Keep something in your pocket or purse that you can take in case of low blood sugar. A packet of sugar, a piece of hard candy, or a small individual box of raisins.

7. **Eating Foods with high Carbohydrate content.** You do not have to stop eating many of the foods that you are used to consuming such as potatoes, rice, or pasta. Just cut down on the portion size as indicated.

8. **Serve your own self at meal time.** Do not allow your wife or family member to fill your plate. They do not like to deny you what they feel is a tasty meal and often overload your plate...And if you are like me, you will eat all of it!

9. **In-between meal Snack.** Chose something that contains little or no Carbohydrates. Cheese, lunch meat, or a piece of the steak left over from dinner. While it may not be the best thing

for your heart, it is best for your diabetes. Being on a low calorie diet, it is doubtful that you would consume harmful amounts of fat anyway.

10. **Don't punish yourself by eating items that do not taste good to you.** I can't stand the taste of low fat salad dressing, and the small amount I eat each day is not enough, in my opinion, to do me great damage. I most likely would stop eating salads if I turned solely to fat free dressings.

11. **Medical advice from a friend or relative.** Everyone has a friend that, in their opinion, are medical experts on every illness, so expect their advice on your condition. You will hear a lot of "Oh one piece of cake won't hurt you". Or, cutting grass isn't doing you any good. You have to lift weights or run for 4 miles at a sustained speed". You be the judge of what you can eat and your ability and necessity for exercise. Chores such as scrubbing and vacuuming the floor, Gardening, patching the roof require energy and burn Carb. and Calories in the process.

12. **Sugar Free Candy.** These candies often contain sorbitol and if a number of pieces are eaten can cause stomach or gas pain. Also, they are not necessarily low in carbohydrates as many contain fructose which is a form of simple sugar.

13. **Spacing your medication.** Take your medication at the same time each day and be sure they are spaced a reasonable period apart.

   I began part time work which brought me home at 1:30 AM at which time I took my "evening" glipizide tablets. Next morning I would take my morning medication upon rising so as not to forget them. This was too close together, and I began to have abdominal pains. After spacing them, the pains ceased.

14. **Check labels when eating out.** Example: I ordered Sugar Free syrup at Perkins restaurant with my pancakes. The cozy cottage sugar free syrup that I use at home is only 9 gr. per 1/4 cup. Perkins is 21 gr. (Here is an added tip: sprinkle a packet of Nutrisweet on the syrup to give it added sweetness.) To avoid the use of syrup all together, Use margarine and Nutrisweet on pancakes and french toast. It might be well to carry your own syrup with you to some restaurants or fast food places.

15. **Fast Food Restaurant.** When ordering hamburgers, or other type sandwiches, remove the top of the the bun or bread. The contents of a sandwich, other than the sauce, usually contain little or no carbohydrates, and may allow you to add a more pleasing item such as a pie, or milk shake.

16. **Bread use.** When purchasing bread for sandwiches, buy the thin sliced if available. This will serve to form the normal sandwich appearance as well as giving you the full taste of the bread. 100% Whole Wheat regular sliced bread has 14 grams of Carb. per slice while the same brand, thin sliced is only 18 gr. for **Two Slices.**

17. Take these charts or this book with you when you leave home. You think that you will remember how many Carbohydrates are in certain foods or Fast Foods, but you will forget. I know I do and I wrote this book! If you don't wish to carry the book, at least tear out the Fast Food Chart and place in your purse or glove compartment of your car.

18. Do take advantage of TV Dinners as a main course for your meals. Here is an excellent opportunity to get suggestions for meals of items that you like. Be sure to check the **total carbohydrates** on each package before you purchase, as they vary greatly. Best of all, they can be stock piled in your freezer and prepared in 6 to 7 minutes. Most of them are low enough in Carbohydrates to allow added vegetable, tomato & cottage cheese salad, and even a dessert. Give them the taste test, and you will find that even a slightly more expensive brand is well worth the extra 50 to 75 cents in taste satisfaction. They are still often less expensive than a home prepared meal. My wife goes along with this as it relieves her of planning and preparing a more elaborate meal.

19. Exercise: This is a personal thing. Do that type of exercise that is most pleasing to you. If you hate it, you will not continue to do it. I find that if I get up in the morning and go out on my bike for 20 min. to 30 minutes immediately after getting out of bed, it is completed before I really have time to think about it. I don't shave, shower, or read the paper. I sometimes vary it with a walk and a walkman so as to not get in a rut, and also before the day's heat gets to the point that it will discourage me.

If possible, find different trails or paths to break up the possability of boredom. Consider a swim in the Municipal pool or a dance with your wife in the garage each evening. It would be good for both of you.

20. Avoid watching long periods of TV. If you are like me, every commercial break is a signal to investigate the refrigerator. I find that while spending time on a computer, I seldom get up for snacks or food. Reading a book or magazine will have the same effect. A night playing aggrevation or dominos with friends may also help, but be sure that any snacks provided are placed on the far side of the table out of reach.

21. Evening Snack Suggestions. I usually have a substantial sized snack around 9:00 or 9:30 each evening. It may consist of a sandwich of Ham, Cheese, or Cotto Salami & Cheese followed by a dish of jello & cool whip. Make it an open faced sandwich and the saved carbohydrates of the one slice of bread will allow you a serving of ice cream in place of the jello.

22. Reducing Carbohydrates by reducing portion sizes. Why use two pieces of bread for a sandwich when one slice will serve as well? Remember, most meats, eggs, cheese, all have near Zero Carbohydrates! Take these as snack items if your blood count is running a little high.

23. Food away from home. If you plan to be away from home for a day or more, don't be afraid to take some items of food that your hosts may not have in the house. My daughters all know that I usually have plenty of jello and cool whip in the house, and this they supply but sometimes they forget, so take along a package or two of Sugar Free Jello, Sugar Free Chocolate Pudding, a couple of containers of Microwave beef stew, or a can of Veg. Barley soup. If you have a small cooler, you may want to include some Cold Cuts, Cheese, or even a little container of Cool whip.

24. **Taking Medication.** If you have trouble taking your Glipizide tablets, I find that chewing them in two or three pieces allow them to go down easily. Surprisingly, they do not have any taste.

25. **Stalling hunger between meals.** I find that a glass of sugar free soft drink, or a cup of hot tea made sweet with a couple of packets of nutrisweet and a dash of cinnamon helps get me to meal time.

EXERCISE - CAN THERE BE TOO MUCH?

Since Phase II Diabetes is basically a disease that occurs mostly in later life, the possibility of over exercise is more unlikely than those in a younger person. Definitely, if you are on insulin, then careful monitoring is only sensible to avoid low blood sugar and the effects of it.

Here again, check with your doctor before taking on any excessive amount of exercise.

It is suggested that you schedule your exercises 1 to 3 hours after a meal as this is the time that your blood glucose is likely to be at its highest point.

Unfortunately, most of us find that we prefer early morning walks, runs, or cycling - especially in the hotter climates in order to beat the heat of the day...Often before we even think of eating breakfast.

Then too, if you are still employed, most of us want to just come home and relax after a days work, and in spite of our best intentions, the exercise loses out.

You may be surprised to know that even up to 24 hours after exercising, your body may require extra food to compensate for the energy used up.

Don't get the idea that I am one that loves to exercise!
Believe me,I hate to waste the fading hours of my life on something so time consuming as walking, biking or lying on the floor in front of a TV and following a VCR tape.

If exercise is productive, then I feel it is not wasted time. Walking the beach or mountain trail, or even spending a day at Disney World on my feet is something I enjoy...Then it is not wasted time.

Oh I know it isn't pleasant when the temperature is over 90 or if there is a raging snow storm out there, but there are alternatives such as indoor equipment, walks in the malls, and yes, even TV morning exercise programs.

This is rather strange that I have this outlook about exercise when my 70 year old wife runs an hour basic exercise class 3 times a week for Seniors. I am afraid to join her class, because I am sure I would embarrass her in front of these older women that can do movements that I would not even consider. In addition she was president of the local Bicycle Club and rides 15 miles every day and sometimes as long as 40 to 50 miles on weekends.

But do it I must, and you should set up a routine for yourself as well. Mowing the lawn or other maintenance jobs, even vacuum the carpet for my wife, at least this is productive.

Then I think of the alternatives if I do not get this exercise, such as poor vision or blindness - sores that will not heal, heart problems, or a stroke, - even kidney failure, all can result from high glucose in the blood and so I push myself out the door for a 3 or 4 mile bike ride, or a half hour walk each day.

SUGGESTED READING

While my book will give you a good working knowledge of what the carbohydrate values are of certain foods, I suggest that you purchase or read: **THE CARBOHYDRATE COUNTER**
      by Corinne T. Netzer
Here you will find a list of Carbohydrate counts for both generic and brand named foods including fast food items that I may not have shown.

The Carbohydrate Counter lists only Carbyhydrate contents. If you wish to know Calorie or other nutrition information, consult your favorite book store or Library.

A Touch of Diabetes, by Lois Jovanovic-Peterson M.D. and Charles M. Peterson M.D. (no relation**ship), & Morton B. Stone.**
This is an up to date informative book for People who have Type II Noninsulin-Dependent Dibetes. It is written in easy to understand language without the complicated jargon of most books of authors of Medical Background.

For information concerning the medical aspect of Phase II diabetes or other forms of diabetes, you may want to obtain the **"American Diabetes Association Complete Guide to Diabetes."**
This book covers all aspects and forms of diabetes including insulin dependency, and childhood forms of the ailment. A very large and expensive book, I suggest you may want to check your local library for a copy.

Calories and Carbohydrates by Barbara Kraus. This book is a dictionary listing of over 8,500 brand names and Basic Foods **with their Calorie and Carbohydrate Counts. This Varies from The Carbohydrate Counter in as much as it has both Calories and Carbohydrates counts while the other has only Carbohydrates shown.**

WHAT TO EAT - WHAT NOT TO EAT

A SPECIAL REMINDER:

ITEMS TO LIMIT SIZE SERVINGS
(high Carb. content)

ITEMS TO USE
(Low Carb. content)

Bagels	Sugar Free Jello
Grapenut Cereal	Cool Whip
Regular Pancake Syrup	Bananas
Ice Cream Shakes or Sundaes	Pears
Fast Food Chicken Sandwiches (fried)	Oranges
Fried Onion Rings	Sugar Free Syrups
Baked Potatoes with Sour Cream	Garden Salad
Potato Skins	Chicken Noodle Soup
Spaghetti (over 1 cup)	Beef, Barley Soup
Red Sauce	TV Dinners
Snack Mixes	Chicken
Regular Soft Drinks	Meats
Large servings of Rice	Eggs
Large servings of Corn	All Vegetables
Fast Food Fish Sandwiches	

PORTION SIZES.

How much is 3 oz. of meat and one gram anyway?

As a rule of thumb, **3 oz. of meat or chicken is the size and thickness of the palm of your hand.**

One Gram is most easily remembered if you take a packet of Nutrisweet and empty it out on the table. **This is one gram!!**

Compare this to a teaspoon of sugar. Not much is it?

Remember, 2 ice cream scoops leveled off equal 1/2 cup.
This same measuring technique can be used for mashed
potatoes, oatmeal, etc.

SICK? IS IT DIABETES OR SOMETHING ELSE?

Once you have been diagnosed as having Phase II diabetes, it is only natural that everytime that you have some other discomfort or ailment that you will blame it on the diabetes.

This is not always true.

Some days you will feel just "Blah" and totally lacking in energy. Other times it is a headache, bodyache, or pains in your stomach.

I once read that even the most healthy of football or baseball players have a day that they just don't feel good, so once in a while those days come around to you.

When I have one of the off days, I usually rely on my blood tester to find out if my sugar is excessively high or low. If not too far from the norm, then it has to be some other cause for the discomfort.

A few months ago I started having abdominal pains, usually in the late evening or during the night which also disrupted my sleep. To begin with it occured maybe once every two or three weeks, then there were periods that it would seem to persist for two or three days at a time and even several times each week.

When I brought this to the attention of my Doctor on a scheduled visit, he sent me to a specialist in Gastroenterology.

Followed were numerous blood tests, stool analysis, upper G.I. X-rays, which all came out negative.

It was first suspected that it might be a return of my peptic ulcer. but this was not the case.

The symptoms, while similar to an ulcer, was different in the that the pain which resembled gas, started in the stomach and progressed down through the intestines and finally ended with a bowel movement.

These episodes, usually lasted for 4 to 5 hours, and then went away.

With no definate diagnosis of any serious problem, I decided to try my own treatment of the disorder by cutting back on the amount of coffee I was drinking, forcing myself to drink water throughout the day.

Then a daily article by a Doctor who answered questions on various subjects was asked about "Irritable Bowel syndrome."

The symptoms he discribed were identical to those that I had been suffering.

In his opinion, this discomfort, while very annoying, does not develop into any other serious malady, and the medical field does not have any specific cure for it.

It seems to be one that affects each individual in different ways, and to relieve it must be through experimentation of eating habits.

I tried to eliminate certain foods that I felt might cause the problem, such as high acid, or spicy foods. For a while the condition would seem to improve and then it would return again dispite the fact that I had eliminated these items.

Some times taking an antacid such as Zantac would help, but only for a period of time.

Then an article written by a doctor was answering a question of a patient who got sick from taking thyroid medication. Since I had been on such a medication for two years I decided to eliminate it for a period of time to see if this could also be my cause of discomfort.

Now after 2 months I have not had another attack of stomach aches even though I have returned to normal eating habits of high acid and spicy foods!

I questioned from the start about any problem with my thyroid glands as I did not have any smptyms of it prior to this time, and after starting taking the pills did not notice any change in my energy level nor metabolism, so I can only assume that the original test was flawed and I should not have been taking the medication anyway.

Self diagnosis and treatment? Doctors don't suggest it and normally I don't try it, but when they throw up their hands and say, "guess you will just have to live with it", then I feel it is justified.

I sometimes think that possibly my diabetic condition which affects the nerve ends may also have a part in it, but then control of my blood sugar is the only answer, and that I am doing anyway.

Sexual Problems

This is a subject that no one wants to bring up nor address, yet it is a known fact that diabetic patients are very often effected by it.

One of the destructive nature of Diabetes is the the effect that it has on nerve endings. Most often publicized is the effect it has on the feet or lower limbs due to poor circulation and sores that may develop on the bottom of the foot without the knowledge of the diabetic because of the lack of feeling in the foot.

This may develop even in cases where blood sugar is considered under control. While my doctor is very pleased with my control results, I still have symptoms that develop from time to time that I know are a direct result from high blood sugar.

Most common for me is the feeling of numbness in my toes. This is not a continuous sensation, but appears occasionally.

For men, another manifestation is ED or Erectal Disfunction. Here again, the damage done to nerve endings comes into play. While this may not be a complete ability to perform, it can be very stressful to the man, and in many cases he will avoid relationships with his wife or partner rather than discuss the problem with her. It could lead to the downfall of marital relations if not confronted directly.

Then too, the cause may be something other than Diabetic.

As men age, they also develop enlargement of the Prostate Gland. This too can cause E.D.

Confide in your Doctor. He may be able to help you with various treatments.

FORMS AND CHARTS

The following pages contain charts and forms for you to use until you get familiar with your daily intake of Carbohydrates. In most cases, you will eat pretty much the same thing for breakfast as you do every day, as well as duplicating lunch and dinner menus.

By use of these forms and charts, you can keep a record for a few weeks to observe what is affecting your blood sugar and you will soon know what foods you should not be eating. Here is an example:

I almost always had two slices of toast and marmalade for breakfast. Then when I checked the chart, I discovered that I could have two eggs, one piece of toast with margarine, and end up with much less carbohydrates than the two pieces of toast and jelly. A much more satisfying breakfast, and a chance for variety.

On the form for the blood count, keep track of it each day at least once a day, preferably the same time, and before you eat. If it suddenly goes up 20 or more points, think what you ate the night before that may have caused it. "Oh yeh, I had popcorn and potato chips. I will have to cut those out or at least a smaller portion." Make note of this in "Comments" and the next time you eat them, see if you have the same reaction.

If you feel you may want more for your use, take them out of the book before you make any entry and run off a few copies on a copy machine.

MINI CARB. & CALORIE CHARTS

The following charts have been reduced in size and show only the Carbohydrate and the Calorie counts for each of the items listed.

This is so that if you wish to have a copy to take with you at all times without carrying the book, it will be a quick reference for you and help you to decide what to eat while away from home.

I took them and placed them back to back and then had them laminated at a local office supply store. This way they can be cut down to pocket size and also will protect them from becoming frayed from handling and use.

Several copies of each page are included so that you can make extra copies for friends and family.

1500 CALORIE DIET
DAILY ALLOWANCE OF CARBOHYDRATES — 155 GRAMS

EVERAGES

ITEM	SERVING SIZE	CARB.	CALORIES
Milk (1%) (Sugar Free)	1 cup	13 grams	110
Hot Chocolate	1 packet	9 grams	50
Diet Soft Drinks (Sugar Sweetened)	8 oz. glass	0 grams	0
Orange Soda	12 oz. can	48 grams	180
Orange Juice	1 Cup	29 grams	120
Grapefruit Juice	1 Cup	24 grams	100
Cranberry Juice Cocktail	8 oz. glass	35 grams	145
Cranapple Juice	8 oz. glass	40 grams	175

1500 CALORIE DIET
DAILY ALLOWANCE OF CARBOHYDRATES - 155 GRAMS

BREADS

ITEM	SERVING SIZE	CARB.	CALORIES
100% whole Wheat Bread	1 Slice	10 grams	50
Pecan Breakfast Bread	1 Slice	14 grams	80
Seeded Rye Bread	1 Slice	14 grams	70
Frozen Waffles	1 waffles	29 grams	190
White Bread	1 Slice	11 grams	50
Rye Crisp	2 Slices	14 grams	70
Soda Crackers	5 Crackers	11 grams	60

1500 CALORIE DIET
DAILY ALLOWANCE OF CARBOHYDRATES — 155 GRAMS

EVERAGES

ITEM	SERVING SIZE	CARB.	CALORIES
Milk (1%) (Sugar Free)	1 cup	13 grams	110
Hot Chocolate	1 packet	9 grams	50
Diet Soft Drinks (Sugar Sweetened)	8 oz. glass	0 grams	0
Orange Soda	12 oz. can	48 grams	180
Orange Juice	1 Cup	29 grams	120
Grapefruit Juice	1 Cup	24 grams	100
Cranberry Juice Cocktail	8 oz. glass	35 grams	145
Cranapple Juice	8 oz. glass	40 grams	175

1500 CALORIE DIET
DAILY ALLOWANCE OF CARBOHYDRATES — 155 GRAMS -

BREADS

ITEM	SERVING SIZE	CARB.	CALORIES
100% whole Wheat Bread	1 Slice	10 grams	50
Pecan Breakfast Bread	1 Slice	14 grams	80
Seeded Rye Bread	1 Slice	14 grams	70
Frozen Waffles	1 waffles	29 grams	190
White Bread	1 Slice	11 grams	50
Rye Crisp	2 Slices	14 grams	70
Soda Crackers	5 Crackers	11 grams	60

1500 CALORIE DIET
DAILY ALLOWANCE OF CARBOHYDRATES — 155 GRAMS

BEVERAGES

ITEM	SERVING SIZE	CARB.	CALORIES
Milk (1%) (Sugar Free)	1 cup	13 grams	110
Hot Chocolate	1 packet	9 grams	50
Diet Soft Drinks (Sugar Sweetened)	8 oz. glass	0 grams	0
Orange Soda	12 oz. can	48 grams	180
Orange Juice	1 Cup	29 grams	120
Grapefruit Juice	1 Cup	24 grams	100
Cranberry Juice Cocktail	8 oz. glass	35 grams	145
Cranapple Juice	8 oz. glass	40 grams	175

1500 CALORIE DIET
DAILY ALLOWANCE OF CARBOHYDRATES - 155 GRAMS

BREADS

ITEM	SERVING SIZE	CARB.	CALORIES
100% whole Wheat Bread	1 Slice	10 grams	50
Pecan Breakfast Bread	1 Slice	14 grams	80
Seeded Rye Bread	1 Slice	14 grams	70
Frozen Waffles	1 waffles	29 grams	190
White Bread	1 Slice	11 grams	50
Rye Crisp	2 Slices	14 grams	70
Soda Crackers	5 Crackers	11 grams	60

1500 CALORIE DIET
DAILY ALLOWANCE OF CARBOHYDRATES — 155 GRAMS

EVERAGES

ITEM	SERVING SIZE	CARB.	CALORIES
Milk (1%) (Sugar Free)	1 cup	13 grams	110
Hot Chocolate	1 packet	9 grams	50
Diet Soft Drinks (Sugar Sweetened)	8 oz. glass	0 grams	0
Orange Soda	12 oz. can	48 grams	180
Orange Juice	1 Cup	29 grams	120
Grapefruit Juice	1 Cup	24 grams	100
Cranberry Juice Cocktail	8 oz. glass	35 grams	145
Cranapple Juice	8 oz. glass	40 grams	175

1500 CALORIE DIET
DAILY ALLOWANCE OF CARBOHYDRATES - 155 GRAMS

BREADS

ITEM	SERVING SIZE	CARB.	CALORIES
100% whole Wheat Bread	1 Slice	10 grams	50
Pecan Breakfast Bread	1 Slice	14 grams	80
Seeded Rye Bread	1 Slice	14 grams	70
Frozen Waffles	1 waffles	29 grams	190
White Bread	1 Slice	11 grams	50
Rye Crisp	2 Slices	14 grams	70
Soda Crackers	5 Crackers	11 grams	60

1500 CALORIE DIET
DAILY ALLOWANCE OF CARBOHYDRATES — 155 GRAMS

BEVERAGES

ITEM	SERVING SIZE	CARB.	CALORIES
Milk (1%) (Sugar Free)	1 cup	13 grams	110
Hot Chocolate	1 packet	9 grams	50
Diet Soft Drinks (Sugar Sweetened)	8 oz. glass	0 grams	0
Orange Soda	12 oz. can	48 grams	180
Orange Juice	1 Cup	29 grams	120
Grapefruit Juice	1 Cup	24 grams	100
Cranberry Juice Cocktail	8 oz. glass	35 grams	145
Cranapple Juice	8 oz. glass	40 grams	175

1500 CALORIE DIET
DAILY ALLOWANCE OF CARBOHYDRATES - 155 GRAMS

BREADS

ITEM	SERVING SIZE	CARB.	CALORIES
100% whole Wheat Bread	1 Slice	10 grams	50
Pecan Breakfast Bread	1 Slice	14 grams	80
Seeded Rye Bread	1 Slice	14 grams	70
Frozen Waffles	1 waffles	29 grams	190
White Bread	1 Slice	11 grams	50
Rye Crisp	2 Slices	14 grams	70
Soda Crackers	5 Crackers	11 grams	60

1500 CALORIE DIET
DAILY ALLOWANCE OF CARBOHYDRATES - 155 GRAMS

CEREALS

ITEM	SERVING SIZE	CARB.	CALORIES
Grape Nuts	1/2 cup	47 grams	200
Honey Bunch of Nuts	3/4 cup	24 grams	130
Cap't Crunch	3/4 cup	23 grams	110
Cheerios	1 cup	22 grams	110
Oatmeal (Cooked)	1 cup	27 grams	150
2% Milk	1/2 cup	6 1/2 grams	150

Milk is shown here as most cereals are eaten with milk added. When consumed with milk, the Carb. and Calorie figures should be added to the cereal contents. Nutritional value of the above should not be determined solely on the above figures, as these figures pertain to use of these products from the diabetic viewpoint. Cereals made from Oats appear to have the lowest amount of Carbohydrates present.

Winton N. Petersen

1500 CALORIE DIET
DAILY ALLOWANCE OF CARBOHYDRATES - 155 GRAMS

DESSERTS AND FRUITS

ITEM	SERVING SIZE	CARB.	CALORIES
Sugar Free Jello	1/2 cup	1 gram	10
Regular Jello	1/2 cup	19 grams	80
Sugar Free Cook & Serve Choc. Pudding	1/2 cup	7 grams	90
Sugar Free Ice Cream Regular-Choc.	1/2 cup	13 grams	90
Almond Ice Cream	1/2 cup	17 grams	170
Cool WhipTopping	2 Tablespoons	2 grams	25
Pears (Canned) Lite	1/2 cup	15 grams	60
Oranges	one	17 grams	75
Banana	one	10 grams	40
Apple	one	21 grams	75

1500 CALORIE DIET
DAILY ALLOWANCE OF CARBOHYDRATES - 155 GRAMS

CEREALS

ITEM	SERVING SIZE	CARB.	CALORIES
Grape Nuts	1/2 cup	47 grams	200
Honey Bunch of Nuts	3/4 cup	24 grams	130
Cap't Crunch	3/4 cup	23 grams	110
Cheerios	1 cup	22 grams	110
Oatmeal (Cooked)	1 cup	27 grams	150
2% Milk	1/2 cup	6 1/2 grams	150

Milk is shown here as most cereals are eaten with milk added. When consumed with milk, the Carb. and Calorie figures should be added to the cereal contents. Nutritional value of the above should not be determined solely on the above figures, as these figures pertain to use of these products from the diabetic viewpoint. Cereals made from Oats appear to have the lowest amount of Carbohydrates present.

Winton N. Petersen

1500 CALORIE DIET
DAILY ALLOWANCE OF CARBOHYDRATES - 155 GRAMS

DESSERTS AND FRUITS

ITEM	SERVING SIZE	CARB.	CALORIES
Sugar Free Jello	1/2 cup	1 gram	10
Regular Jello	1/2 cup	19 grams	80
Sugar Free Cook & Serve Choc. Pudding	1/2 cup	7 grams	90
Sugar Free Ice Cream Regular-Choc.	1/2 cup	13 grams	90
Almond Ice Cream	1/2 cup	17 grams	170
Cool WhipTopping	2 Tablespoons	2 grams	25
Pears (Canned) Lite	1/2 cup	15 grams	60
Oranges	one	17 grams	75
Banana	one	10 grams	40
Apple	one	21 grams	75

1500 CALORIE DIET
DAILY ALLOWANCE OF CARBOHYDRATES - 155 GRAMS

CEREALS

ITEM	SERVING SIZE	CARB.	CALORIES
Grape Nuts	1/2 cup	47 grams	200
Honey Bunch of Nuts	3/4 cup	24 grams	130
Cap't Crunch	3/4 cup	23 grams	110
Cheerios	1 cup	22 grams	110
Oatmeal (Cooked)	1 cup	27 grams	150
2% Milk	1/2 cup	6 1/2 grams	150

Milk is shown here as most cereals are eaten with milk added. When consumed with milk, the Carb. and Calorie figures should be added to the cereal contents. Nutritional value of the above should not be determined solely on the above figures, as these figures pertain to use of these products from the diabetic viewpoint. Cereals made from Oats appear to have the lowest amount of Carbohydrates present.

1500 CALORIE DIET
DAILY ALLOWANCE OF CARBOHYDRATES - 155 GRAMS

DESSERTS AND FRUITS

ITEM	SERVING SIZE	CARB.	CALORIES
Sugar Free Jello	1/2 cup	1 gram	10
Regular Jello	1/2 cup	19 grams	80
Sugar Free Cook & Serve Choc. Pudding	1/2 cup	7 grams	90
Sugar Free Ice Cream	1/2 cup	13 grams	90
Regular-Choc. Almond Ice Cream	1/2 cup	17 grams	170
Cool WhipTopping	2 Tablespoons	2 grams	25
Pears (Canned) Lite	1/2 cup	15 grams	60
Oranges	one	17 grams	75
Banana	one	10 grams	40
Apple	one	21 grams	75

1500 CALORIE DIET
DAILY ALLOWANCE OF CARBOHYDRATES - 155 GRAMS

CEREALS

ITEM	SERVING SIZE	CARB.	CALORIES
Grape Nuts	1/2 cup	47 grams	200
Honey Bunch of Nuts	3/4 cup	24 grams	130
Cap't Crunch	3/4 cup	23 grams	110
Cheerios	1 cup	22 grams	110
Oatmeal (Cooked)	1 cup	27 grams	150
2% Milk	1/2 cup	6 1/2 grams	150

Milk is shown here as most cereals are eaten with milk added. When consumed with milk, the Carb. and Calorie figures should be added to the cereal contents. Nutritional value of the above should not be determined solely on the above figures, as these figures pertain to use of these products from the diabetic viewpoint. Cereals made from Oats appear to have the lowest amount of Carbohydrates present.

1500 CALORIE DIET
DAILY ALLOWANCE OF CARBOHYDRATES - 155 GRAMS

DESSERTS AND FRUITS

ITEM	SERVING SIZE	CARB.	CALORIES
Sugar Free Jello	1/2 cup	1 gram	10
Regular Jello	1/2 cup	19 grams	80
Sugar Free Cook & Serve Choc. Pudding	1/2 cup	7 grams	90
Sugar Free Ice Cream Regular-Choc.	1/2 cup	13 grams	90
Almond Ice Cream	1/2 cup	17 grams	170
Cool WhipTopping	2 Tablespoons	2 grams	25
Pears (Canned) Lite	1/2 cup	15 grams	60
Oranges	one	17 grams	75
Banana	one	10 grams	40
Apple	one	21 grams	75

1500 CALORIE DIET
DAILY ALLOWANCE OF CARBOHYDRATES - 155 GRAMS

CEREALS

ITEM	SERVING SIZE	CARB.	CALORIES
Grape Nuts	1/2 cup	47 grams	200
Honey Bunch of Nuts	3/4 cup	24 grams	130
Cap't Crunch	3/4 cup	23 grams	110
Cheerios	1 cup	22 grams	110
Oatmeal (Cooked)	1 cup	27 grams	150
2% Milk	1/2 cup	6 1/2 grams	150

Milk is shown here as most cereals are eaten with milk added. When consumed with milk, the Carb. and Calorie figures should be added to the cereal contents. Nutritional value of the above should not be determined solely on the above figures, as these figures pertain to use of these products from the diabetic viewpoint. Cereals made from Oats appear to have the lowest amount of Carbohydrates present.

1500 CALORIE DIET
DAILY ALLOWANCE OF CARBOHYDRATES - 155 GRAMS

DESSERTS AND FRUITS

ITEM	SERVING SIZE	CARB.	CALORIES
Sugar Free Jello	1/2 cup	1 gram	10
Regular Jello	1/2 cup	19 grams	80
Sugar Free Cook & Serve Choc. Pudding	1/2 cup	7 grams	90
Sugar Free Ice Cream Regular-Choc.	1/2 cup	13 grams	90
Almond Ice Cream	1/2 cup	17 grams	170
Cool WhipTopping	2 Tablespoons	2 grams	25
Pears (Canned) Lite	1/2 cup	15 grams	60
Oranges	one	17 grams	75
Banana	one	10 grams	40
Apple	one	21 grams	75

1500 CALORIE DIET
DAILY ALLOWANCE OF CARBOHYDRATES - 155 GRAMS

FAST FOODS

ITEM	SERVING SIZE	CARB.	CALORIES

MC DONALD'S

BREAKFST ITEMS

ITEM	SERVING SIZE	CARB.	CALORIES
Breakfast Biscuit (plain)	one	32 grams	290
Breakfast Biscuit w/sausage	one	33 grams	470
Pancakes w/syrup	three	100 grams	570

MEALTIME ITEMS

ITEM	SERVING SIZE	CARB.	CALORIES
Big Mac	one	45 grams	560
Qtr Pounder	one	37 grams	420
Chicken Mcnuggets	six	15 grams	290
French Fries	small	26 grams	210
Apple pie	one	34 grams	260
Ice Cream Shake	small	60 grams	360
Sundae (Choc.)	one	52 grams	340
Garden Salad	one	7 grams	35
Ranch Dressing	one pkt	10 grams	230

1500 CALORIE DIET
DAILY ALLOWANCE OF CARBOHYDRATES - 155 GRAMS

ITEM	SERVING SIZE	CARB.	CALORIES
BURGER KING			
Croissan'wich	one	25 grams	530
Hashbrowns	one pc.	25 grams	220
Whopper	one	45 grams	630
Chicken Sand.	one	54 grams	700
Onion Rings	small	41 grams	310
ARBY'S			
Curly fries	Regular	38 grams	300
Roast Beef Sand.	Regular	33 grams	388
Fish Sand.	one	50 grams	529
orsey Sauce	one Tblsp.	2 grams	60
Baked Potato/sour cream	one	85 grams	578
Cheese Cake	one slice	23 grams	320
WENDY'S			
Jr. Bacon/Cheeseburger	one	34 grams	380
Hamburger, plain	one	31 grams	360
Chilli	8 oz.	21 grams	227
Baked PotatoBacon & Cheese	one small	78 grams	380

1500 CALORIE DIET
DAILY ALLOWANCE OF CARBOHYDRATES - 155 GRAMS

ITEM	SERVING SIZE	CARB.	CALORIES
MC DONALD'S			
BREAKFST ITEMS			
Breakfast Biscuit (plain)	one	32 grams	290
Breakfast Biscuit w/sausage	one	33 grams	470
Pancakes w/syrup	three	100 grams	570
MEALTIME ITEMS			
Big Mac	one	45 grams	560
Qtr Pounder	one	37 grams	420
Chicken Mcnuggets	six	15 grams	290
French Fries	small	26 grams	210
Apple pie	one	34 grams	260
Ice Cream Shake	small	60 grams	360
Sundae (Choc.)	one	52 grams	340
Garden Salad	one	7 grams	35
Ranch Dressing	one pkt	10 grams	230

1500 CALORIE DIET
DAILY ALLOWANCE OF CARBOHYDRATES - 155 GRAMS

ITEM	SERVING SIZE	CARB.	CALORIES

BURGER KING

ITEM	SERVING SIZE	CARB.	CALORIES
Croissan'wich	one	25 grams	530
Hashbrowns	one pc.	25 grams	220
Whopper	one	45 grams	630
Chicken Sand.	one	54 grams	700
Onion Rings	small	41 grams	310

ARBY'S

ITEM	SERVING SIZE	CARB.	CALORIES
Curly fries	Regular	38 grams	300
Roast Beef Sand.	Regular	33 grams	388
Fish Sand.	one	50 grams	529
orsey Sauce	one Tblsp.	2 grams	60
Baked Potato/sour cream	one	85 grams	578
Cheese Cake	one slice	23 grams	320

WENDY'S

ITEM	SERVING SIZE	CARB.	CALORIES
Jr. Bacon/Cheeseburger	one	34 grams	380
Hamburger, plain	one	31 grams	360
Chilli	8 oz.	21 grams	227
Baked PotatoBacon & Cheese	one small	78 grams	380

1500 CALORIE DIET
DAILY ALLOWANCE OF CARBOHYDRATES - 155 GRAMS

ITEM	SERVING SIZE	CARB.	CALORIES

MC DONALD'S

BREAKFST ITEMS

ITEM	SERVING SIZE	CARB.	CALORIES
Breakfast Biscuit (plain)	one	32 grams	290
Breakfast Biscuit w/sausage	one	33 grams	470
Pancakes w/syrup	three	100 grams	570

MEALTIME ITEMS

ITEM	SERVING SIZE	CARB.	CALORIES
Big Mac	one	45 grams	560
Qtr Pounder	one	37 grams	420
Chicken Mcnuggets	six	15 grams	290
French Fries	small	26 grams	210
Apple pie	one	34 grams	260
Ice Cream Shake	small	60 grams	360
Sundae (Choc.)	one	52 grams	340
Garden Salad	one	7 grams	35
Ranch Dressing	one pkt	10 grams	230

1500 CALORIE DIET
DAILY ALLOWANCE OF CARBOHYDRATES - 155 GRAMS

ITEM	SERVING SIZE	CARB.	CALORIES
BURGER KING			
Croissan'wich	one	25 grams	530
Hashbrowns	one pc.	25 grams	220
Whopper	one	45 grams	630
Chicken Sand.	one	54 grams	700
Onion Rings	small	41 grams	310
ARBY'S			
Curly fries	Regular	38 grams	300
Roast Beef Sand.	Regular	33 grams	388
Fish Sand.	one	50 grams	529
orsey Sauce	one Tblsp.	2 grams	60
Baked Potato/ sour cream	one	85 grams	578
Cheese Cake	one slice	23 grams	320
WENDY'S			
Jr. Bacon/Cheeseburger	one	34 grams	380
Hamburger, plain	one	31 grams	360
Chilli	8 oz.	21 grams	227
Baked PotatoBacon & Cheese	one small	78 grams	380

1500 CALOIRE DIET
DAILY ALLOWANCE OF CARBOHYDRATES - 155 GRAMS

ITEM	SERVING SIZE	CARB.	CALORIES

MC DONALD'S

BREAKFST ITEMS

ITEM	SERVING SIZE	CARB.	CALORIES
Breakfast Biscuit (plain)	one	32 grams	290
Breakfast Biscuit w/sausage	one	33 grams	470
Pancakes w/syrup	three	100 grams	570

MEALTIME ITEMS

ITEM	SERVING SIZE	CARB.	CALORIES
Big Mac	one	45 grams	560
Qtr Pounder	one	37 grams	420
Chicken Mcnuggets	six	15 grams	290
French Fries	small	26 grams	210
Apple pie	one	34 grams	260
Ice Cream Shake	small	60 grams	360
Sundae (Choc.)	one	52 grams	340
Garden Salad	one	7 grams	35
Ranch Dressing	one pkt	10 grams	230

1500 CALORIE DIET
DAILY ALLOWANCE OF CARBOHYDRATES - 155 GRAMS

ITEM	SERVING SIZE	CARB.	CALORIES
BURGER KING			
Croissan'wich	one	25 grams	530
Hashbrowns	one pc.	25 grams	220
Whopper	one	45 grams	630
Chicken Sand.	one	54 grams	700
Onion Rings	small	41 grams	310
ARBY'S			
Curly fries	Regular	38 grams	300
Roast Beef Sand.	Regular	33 grams	388
Fish Sand.	one	50 grams	529
orsey Sauce	one Tblsp.	2 grams	60
Baked Potato/ sour cream	one	85 grams	578
Cheese Cake	one slice	23 grams	320
WENDY'S			
Jr. Bacon/Cheeseburger	one	34 grams	380
Hamburger, plain	one	31 grams	360
Chilli	8 oz.	21 grams	227
Baked PotatoBacon & Cheese	one small	78 grams	380

1500 CALORIE DIET
DAILY ALLOWANCE OF CARBOHYDRATES - 155 GRAMS

ITEM	SERVING SIZE	CARB.	CALORIES
MC DONALD'S			
BREAKFST ITEMS			
Breakfast Biscuit (plain)	one	32 grams	290
Breakfast Biscuit w/sausage	one	33 grams	470
Pancakes w/syrup	three	100 grams	570
MEALTIME ITEMS			
Big Mac	one	45 grams	560
Qtr Pounder	one	37 grams	420
Chicken Mcnuggets	six	15 grams	290
French Fries	small	26 grams	210
Apple pie	one	34 grams	260
Ice Cream Shake	small	60 grams	360
Sundae (Choc.)	one	52 grams	340
Garden Salad	one	7 grams	35
Ranch Dressing	one pkt	10 grams	230

1500 CALORIE DIET
DAILY ALLOWANCE OF CARBOHYDRATES - 155 GRAMS

ITEM	SERVING SIZE	CARB.	CALORIES
BURGER KING			
Croissan'wich	one	25 grams	530
Hashbrowns	one pc.	25 grams	220
Whopper	one	45 grams	630
Chicken Sand.	one	54 grams	700
Onion Rings	small	41 grams	310
ARBY'S			
Curly fries	Regular	38 grams	300
Roast Beef Sand.	Regular	33 grams	388
Fish Sand.	one	50 grams	529
orsey Sauce	one Tblsp.	2 grams	60
Baked Potato/ sour cream	one	85 grams	578
Cheese Cake	one slice	23 grams	320
WENDY'S			
Jr. Bacon/Cheeseburger	one	34 grams	380
Hamburger, plain	one	31 grams	360
Chilli	8 oz.	21 grams	227
Baked PotatoBacon & Cheese	one small	78 grams	380

BLANK FORMS

DATE_____DAY_____

FOOD EATEN   **CARBHYDRATES**   **CALORIES**

   BREAKFAST

   SNACK

   LUNCH

   SNACK

   DINNER

   SNACK

BLOOD TEST _____ before meal   TIME TAKEN_____

DATE_____DAY_____

FOOD EATEN	CARBHYDRATES	CALORIES
BREAKFAST		
SNACK		
LUNCH		
SNACK		
DINNER		
SNACK		

BLOOD TEST _____ before meal   TIME TAKEN_____

DATE_____DAY_____

FOOD EATEN   CARBOHYDRATES   CALORIESDATE_____DAY_____

FOOD EATEN   CARBHYDRATES   CALORIES

   BREAKFAST

   SNACK

   LUNCH

   SNACK

   DINNER

   SNACK

BLOOD TEST _____ before meal   TIME TAKEN_____

DATE_____DAY_____

FOOD EATEN **CARBHYDRATES** **CALORIES**

BREAKFAST

SNACK

LUNCH

SNACK

DINNER

SNACK

BLOOD TEST _____ before meal **TIME TAKEN_____**

DATE_____DAY_____

FOOD EATEN   **CARBHYDRATES**   **CALORIES**

    BREAKFAST

    SNACK

    LUNCH

    SNACK

    DINNER

    SNACK

BLOOD TEST _____ before meal   TIME TAKEN_____

MONTH_____

DATE	TIME	BLOOD COUNT	COMENTS
_____	_____	_____	_____
_____	_____	_____	_____
_____	_____	_____	_____
_____	_____	_____	_____
_____	_____	_____	_____
_____	_____	_____	_____
_____	_____	_____	_____
_____	_____	_____	_____
_____	_____	_____	_____
_____	_____	_____	_____
_____	_____	_____	_____
_____	_____	_____	_____
_____	_____	_____	_____

AVERAGE TOTAL FOR MONTH _____

MONTH_____

DATE	TIME	BLOOD COUNT	COMENTS
_____	_____	_____	_____
_____	_____	_____	_____
_____	_____	_____	_____
_____	_____	_____	_____
_____	_____	_____	_____
_____	_____	_____	_____
_____	_____	_____	_____
_____	_____	_____	_____
_____	_____	_____	_____
_____	_____	_____	_____
_____	_____	_____	_____
_____	_____	_____	_____
_____	_____	_____	_____

AVERAGE TOTAL FOR MONTH _____

Winton N. Petersen

MONTH_____

DATE	TIME	BLOOD COUNT	COMENTS
_____	_____	_____	_____
_____	_____	_____	_____
_____	_____	_____	_____
_____	_____	_____	_____
_____	_____	_____	_____
_____	_____	_____	_____
_____	_____	_____	_____
_____	_____	_____	_____
_____	_____	_____	_____
_____	_____	_____	_____
_____	_____	_____	_____
_____	_____	_____	_____
_____	_____	_____	_____

AVERAGE TOTAL FOR MONTH   _____

MONTH_____

DATE	TIME	BLOOD COUNT	COMENTS
_____	_____	_____	_____
_____	_____	_____	_____
_____	_____	_____	_____
_____	_____	_____	_____
_____	_____	_____	_____
_____	_____	_____	_____
_____	_____	_____	_____
_____	_____	_____	_____
_____	_____	_____	_____
_____	_____	_____	_____
_____	_____	_____	_____
_____	_____	_____	_____
_____	_____	_____	_____

AVERAGE TOTAL FOR MONTH _____

Winton N. Petersen

MONTH_____

DATE	TIME	BLOOD COUNT	COMENTS
_____	_____	_____	_____
_____	_____	_____	_____
_____	_____	_____	_____
_____	_____	_____	_____
_____	_____	_____	_____
_____	_____	_____	_____
_____	_____	_____	_____
_____	_____	_____	_____
_____	_____	_____	_____
_____	_____	_____	_____
_____	_____	_____	_____
_____	_____	_____	_____
_____	_____	_____	_____

AVERAGE TOTAL FOR MONTH _____

About the Author

The son of two diabetic parents, the Author was considered at risk for contracting the disease.

A walking mail carrier for 15 years in the Florida sun & heat possibly saved him from becoming diabetic earlier due to the great amount of physical exercise involved, but one year after retirement in 1984 on a visit to a VA clinic, he was diagnosed as having Phase II diabetes.

After retirement from the Postal Service, He took more sedentary employment, first as a Real Estate Salesperson, and the for the past 3 years part time employment for Nielsen Media Research.....Both desk jobs.

As a result, his blood Sugar count continued to increase and he realized that he had to take more drastic action in order keep his condition under control.

Counting CARBOHYDRATES was the answer for him.

Written in laymen's language it gives the Patient's Point of View, and the resulting positive results.

www.ingramcontent.com/pod-product-compliance
Lightning Source LLC
Chambersburg PA
CBHW080417290526
45791CB00008BA/2311